£2.85 EHCM

FAMILY PLANNING DROP-OUTS RECONSIDERED

A Critical Review of Research and Research Findings

by

Philip Kreager

International Planned Parenthood Federation
18-20 Lower Regent Street, London SW1Y 4PW

November 1977

TABLE OF CONTENTS

This review constituted one of the background papers of the IPPF Social Science Working Party's meeting of June 1977, Colombo, Sri Lanka. The views expressed by the author are based on his analysis of the research literature, and should not be taken to represent the social science policy of IPPF. The latter is under discussion at the time the present publication goes into print.

The full annotated bibliography and further details of the research on which this publication is based are available in the IPPF Central Library.

Any queries, comments and requests should be directed to:

Dr. Angela Molnos
IPPF Social Sciences Adviser
International Planned Parenthood Federation
18-20 Lower Regent Street
London SW1Y 4PW
England

ISBN 0 86089 010 4

FOREWORD

The question of "drop-outs" in the field of family planning services is one on which a large number of publications appeared over the last decade. More recently there has been an increasing demand for somebody to pull together all the findings and tell us what we really know about this problem and what we don't. As far as we know, the present work by Philip Kreager is the first critical bibliography and assessment of scientific materials related to family planning discontinuation rates. His analysis leads to important conclusions for future research and evaluation efforts in this area. The author is less explicit in making recommendations for family planning programmes. This is partly due to the confined practical applicability of available research findings and partly to the fact that one is reluctant to make any practical suggestion for improvement other than in relation to a concrete programme. Despite these two limitations, I have singled out five major implications from his review and expanded upon them from what might be the standpoint of programme planners and programme administrators.

First, planners and administrators should treat 'discontinuation rates' not as an undesirable phenomenon but as a regular and foreseeable feature of all programmes. So far 'drop-outs' have been considered 'resisters'. This negative connotation makes administrators and researchers ask some misplaced questions like: "Is it the programme's fault?" "Is it the client's fault?" Such questions stand in the way of a thorough understanding of what really happens. They obscure the fact that some segments of 'drop-outs' constitute a success story for the programme. In fact, many of those who are recorded under this concept are doing exactly what programmes want them to do: they have a planned child or practise birth control with another programme or on their own. Yet other clients have never seriously accepted the practice of family planning and therefore should not be considered 'drop-outs'. The drop-out situation of each programme has to be examined in relation to its definition of 'acceptor'. Obviously the looser the concept 'acceptor', the higher will be the drop-out rate. Both concepts need tightening up. Once it is recognized that discontinuation rates can be indicators of both, failure as well as success, the usual under-reporting of discontinuation in clinic records will also improve. The exclusively negative connotation of 'drop-outs', however, can only be dispelled by an ongoing element of self-evaluation of programmes. Such evaluation should include periodical follow-up of those who abandoned the programme.

Secondly, there is sufficient evidence in the scientific literature pointing to the crucial importance of the first contact with the client. In general it is fair to assume that the initial stages of the adoption of family planning practice by each client are the decisive ones. The longer a client practises family planning the more likely she/he is to continue. Although the importance of the first contact and of the initial stages are known to most programme personnel, programmes do not always cater for the special needs of new clients. Hence the inflated numbers of those 'drop-outs' who never began to practise family planning in earnest. One reason for failing to apply what is well known, might lie with the policy pursued by some programmes. Those programmes which measure their success by the "number of births prevented" are less likely to cater for the individual needs of new clients than programmes which have a policy to assist clients in making free decisions one way or the other about their own fertility. Paradoxically, in the long run the latter programmes are more likely to retain clients and to "prevent births".

The counselling effort on the first contact has to be very careful as well as intensive. It has to compensate for any negative reactions linked with the initial medical check-up which can be off-putting. The latter should be organized in a way which is least offensive to the individual client (given her/his cultural background and individual situation). Unless the counsellor addresses himself to the client's real problems when the client first learns about contraceptives, those problems will be aggravated and become chronical. The counsellor - the family planning educator - must therefore know how to find out from clients what are their real problems. This requirement implies that programme personnel in contact with new clients must have a strong client-orientated attitude (as opposed to a programme-orientated one) and be able to withhold any preconceived ideas of their own in order to understand the client's points of view and needs. They must also be trained in adequate interviewing techniques.

Physical complications are to be expected for many users of the IUD and pill. If these are anticipated and explained at the outset by someone who knows the client's socio-cultural, personal and psychological background, then the client will be more likely to deal with such complications in a matter of fact way and less likely to abandon the whole idea of family planning because of fear of side-effects.

Initial counselling should not oversell any given contraceptive method but on the contrary explain the major advantages and disadvantages of each. Personnel have to be specifically trained not to push one method of contraception over another, but to remain objective and help the client to make up her/his own mind. Obviously the precondition is that the programme does offer genuine alternatives to suit not only the particular physical requirements of clients, but also to suit socio-cultural and individual conditions, as well as particular psychological needs. A choice of methods is also necessary in order to retain some of those who otherwise would drop-out because of dissatisfaction with a particular method. As the author points out "a drop-out is more likely to try another method than make a second attempt at the same method."

The extreme importance of the first stages also requires a thorough briefing of all personnel on these problems and not only of those selected to counsel new clients. It is essential to make sure that the client does not receive any contradictory information or advice from different staff members with whom she comes into contact.

Thirdly, there is an urgent need to review programmes critically from the point of view of the community in which they operate and to adapt each programme to the socio-cultural background of the clients served. This call to adapt programmes to local conditions and to local socio-cultural requirements is not new. The research evidence contained in this review forcibly re-states it.[1] There might be several explanations why a substantial part of family planning services has failed to take into account the cultural background and ended up by reinforcing cultural barriers. Whatever the explanations might be, the difficulty to involve the true representatives of the community in programme planning and evaluation, the pressures on the programme administrator to show quantitative results (number of continuing acceptors, births prevented) rather than qualitative success (satisfaction among clients and the community), one can only reiterate the warning: to ignore the local culture is in the long run counterproductive and very harmful to everyone involved.

Thorough local knowledge of language, customs, social networks, attitudes, etc. is required to plan new programmes and to improve existing ones. The most relevant questions will have to be answered by the people themselves. In general programmes should periodically be revised in order to assess how their clients are affected by travelling distances, waiting times, medical and other procedures, and the attitude of staff. The answer in each case will depend on the socio-cultural background of the clients served. One can only stress again and again the

---

1 The author laid an even greater stress on this point in the first version of this work which had to be reduced in size. We expect to publish his original chapter which dealt with the cultural aspects of research on discontinuation rates at a future date.

almost classic recommendations S.C. Scrimshaw (290) made for an Ecuatorian clinic. Most of the answers to problems of programme operations can be given only locally. For instance, whether the husband should receive counselling together with his wife; what are the various types of prevalent sexual relationships to which different contraceptive methods are suited (such as "visiting unions"); which are the relevant reference groups which exert influence and which have to be involved in the programme planning. In dealing with clients and drop-outs socio-cultural and psychological factors have to be taken into account as seriously as medical factors.

Fourthly, special attention should be paid to examining and improving the ability of clinic staff to respect and serve the client's cultural and individual needs. Obviously, if programmes have to become client-orientated and cater for clients' socio-cultural and psychological needs then all will hinge on the selection and training of staff.[2] Only such personnel who have sensitivity, common sense, non-authoritarian attitudes, a thorough knowledge of the local language and culture should be selected. They should be people to whom clients enjoy talking about their concerns and hopes.

From time to time programmes have to be evaluated as to whether there are recurring problems with attitudes and behaviour of staff which are systematically affecting clients' reactions to programmes. In other words, staff/client interactions have to be monitored, periodically revised, improvements suggested and implemented. This means periodical training of staff. Certainly staff should not be allowed to learn the hard way about the client's cultural background, namely through initial misunderstandings, tensions or clashes with clients.

---

2 See: Selection of Field Personnel; Training of Field Personnel in: A. MOLNOS, Cultural Source Materials for Family Planning in East Africa, Nairobi, East African Publishing House for the Institute of African Studies, University of Nairobi, Vol.II, 1972, p.56 and 58.

Attention has to be drawn to the programme implications of the local culture before staff begin to work with clients. Even personnel belonging to the same culture have to be helped to see all the implications from the clients' point of view. Programme personnel have to learn elementary techniques of research to be able to find out on an ongoing basis the information needed for their work.[3]

Fifthly, the evidence shows that all this can only be achieved through sound and constructive co-operation between programme planners, administrators, programme personnel on the one hand and researchers on the other. If so little of the mass of available research is practically useful, this is partly due to the fact that administrators do not place sufficiently strong demands on researchers to serve programmes. Most programme people have a good grasp of the local situation. They should not allow researchers to plan their research on wrong assumptions or to waste resources on finding out the obvious. There is no reason why administrators should accept banal or stereotype explanations as research findings. Programme planners and administrators should request that researchers have a thorough knowledge of the local culture and socio-economic conditions before starting their research. Programme planners and administrators should use researchers with local knowledge to incorporate an ongoing evaluation element in the design of family planning programmes. Such evaluation should extend to that segment of acceptors who will discontinue. (As said, numbers and characteristics of drop-outs can be anticipated). Provisions have to be made to be able to locate and follow-up a representative portion of future drop-outs (e.g. by registering not only personal address, but also a contact person's address). The evaluation scheme has to take into account the values and goals of the community in which the programme operates.

---

3 See: Research and Action: Guidelines for Outside Innovators with Special Reference to Family Planning Field Workers in: A. Molnos, op. cit., Vol. 11, p. 380.

Researchers should be used to design experimental schemes such as testing different types of educational approaches.

The implications of this critical examination of the literature on drop-outs are relevant to designing and organizing new research approaches. Research planners and research workers will be interested to study this review closely. The major recommendations for research which arise from this wealth of critical data are the need to revise current concepts of discontinuation, to study "drop-outs" within their socio-cultural context and less in relation to contraceptive methods, and finally to develop new research approaches and techniques accordingly.

The current concept of discontinuation ('drop-outs') ignores the complexities of method shifts and interruptions and the diverse reasons underlying apparently identical behaviour. It covers therefore such a great variety of cases as to become nearly meaningless. This concept along with other categorizations such as "motivated/non-motivated", "medical/non-medical reasons for discontinuation", "wanted/unwanted pregnancy", "urban/rural groups", etc. are the product of a research tradition dominated by demographic studies, clinical statistics and KAP surveys. Most of these concepts heavily overlap with their alleged opposites. They have come into use because the accurate measures imposed by the research tradition require clear-cut concepts which can be manipulated quantitatively. However, such concepts are stereotypes established a priori before analysing the concrete background. Research findings based on them have little explanatory value.

Past research "on and around" the drop-out problem (as the author aptly expresses it) has its merits: it developed simple and practicable record-keeping and evaluation techniques; and it has shown the limits of external (i.e. non-contextual) measurements, thus leading to the current concern about the socio-cultural context in which family planning programmes operate. The author calls for an increased use of local, cultural, "contextual" information to understand the drop-out problem in each concrete setting. It is not enough to add simply a couple of questions on "culture" or to use local personnel for research. What is needed is an entirely new research approach. However, local information is often overwhelming because of its quantity and anecdotal character. A first priority should be to develop guidelines on how to collect, select, process and use such materials. The other danger of cultural research is that of re-inventing the ordinary.[4] A discovery made by the researcher might be just a commonsensical fact for a local person or even for programme staff. In order to prevent this happening, before starting to plan the research the researcher has to make a thorough study of the available literature on the area and exploit all other unobtrusive ways, such as daily contacts, to get acquainted with the particular culture and community. Finally, the research design has to be developed, checked, and the research conducted in close co-operation with those who know most about the area, ultimately with the people themselves among whom the research will be conducted.[5] New research designs can be developed in order to tap systematically the knowledge of those people within the community who have most information on clients who discontinued the practice of family planning.

The author suggests that future 'drop-out' research should concentrate on the following areas: on the question of how people drop out from programmes, on short term discontinuation (including type of circumstances of initial use), on potential clients who come only once but without accepting any method, on changes in contraceptive methods, on post-termination events, on clinic-related factors affecting continuation, on the question to what

---

4 See: From Attitude Research to Cultural Information, in: A. Molnos, op.cit., Vol.I, p.56.

5 B.L. Hall: Participatory Research: An Approach for Change. Convergence, Vol.VIII, 1975, No.2, 24-31.

extent medical complaints overlap with service-related complaints. The overall recommendation is that research designs should become more client-orientated and less method-orientated. Single method studies should be avoided, since their findings are more misleading than helpful.

In reviewing the literature the author found that too often essential information is missing in research reports. Researchers should be aware of the fact that details of how the research was conducted are essential for the reader to understand fully the meaning and the value of the findings and ultimately to utilize them.

Research reports should always make explicit the following information: objective and hypotheses, period of research with dates, exact geographical area, details of sample, details of interviewing, other data collecting techniques, data processing, definitions of concepts, number and type of research staff used, their degree of familiarity with local language and culture. Finally, all specific methodological experiences, failures and successes, should be reported as they are invaluable to future researchers.

According to Kreager "The limits of our knowledge on the subject are the limits of the traditions of research that have been applied to or rather, around the problem". Hopefully there will be many researchers who as a result of reading this publication, will set out to establish new research designs in order to overcome restrictive research traditions. The ultimate aim of the researchers should be to identify the true 'drop-outs' and to make a substantial contribution to the practitioners' efforts to reduce their numbers. A reduction of discontinuation rates is required not only in order to prevent considerable wastage of resources and increase programme cost-effectiveness. Every dissatisfied, disappointed or distressed user means also psychological and social costs which it is our urgent responsibility to reduce.

I wish to express our thanks to the author for performing the valuable work and the task of making it accessible to a broader readership.

London, November, 1977

Dr. Angela Molnos
IPPF Social Sciences Adviser

PREFACE BY THE AUTHOR

There is an evident need to identify the social situations and processes which discourage and even drive away users of family planning services. Yet anyone familiar with this issue can only be impressed by two facts: first, the considerable number of writings which touch in some way on the problem; and second, the difficulty of applying the literature to the practical realities of family planning programmes. This review is based on the premise that studies of discontinuation need to be integrated in order to see what direction they can give to programme activities. The limits of our knowledge on the subject are the limits of the traditions of research that have been applied to or rather around the problem.

The picture we have gained to date of drop-outs is fragmentary; it typically consists of a number of user attributes (socio-demographic characteristics and stereotyped reasons for discontinuing a first method) and a few clinic variables. The selection of these categories reflects research conventions more than the indigenous values and conditions which shape users' actions. Discontinuation emerges as a peripheral topic in each successive wave of population research. Most of the literature ostensibly about discontinuation skirts round the personal, cultural and social factors that make up programme-user-method interaction.

It seems impossible to understand 'drop-outs' in isolation, that is without considering them a normal part of patterns of contraceptive continuation and discontinuation. The physiological effects of methods such as the IUD and oral contraceptives, the differing needs of women at different periods of their life cycle, and the diverse influence of cultures make it inevitable that there are several such patterns in any contracepting population. Thus, we should expect an appropriate concept of discontinuation to vary with reference to specific populations according to local modes of thought and action, and to allow for several variations such as the timing, number and kinds of methods used.

This review of the literature on family planning drop-outs is confined to Asian, African and Latin American materials, except where notable methodological developments are concerned. Some European and American studies have been included because they contain interesting programme innovations or rarely asked questions that may be relevant to the problem. An attempt has been made at complete coverage; however the varying availability of published and unpublished sources must cast doubt on this. In addition, it should be noted that a number of articles, perhaps ten per cent of those included in the bibliography, were not available at the time of writing. Bibliographic entries are cited in the text by number in parentheses. A few further references are made in the course of argument to articles which do not belong in a bibliography of discontinuation; these are indicated by footnotes. A more extensive bibliography, with annotations of eighty of the more important entries, is available in the IPPF Central Office Library.

There are four important acknowledgements. Dr. Angela Molnos, Social Sciences Adviser to IPPF, encouraged a review of the literature on this topic, and made helpful comments at several stages of the work. Catherine Howell's editorial criticism improved the clarity and readability of the text. I am indebted to the librarians of the IPPF Central Office Library on numerous points of advice and guidance. The several revisions of the manuscript were typed by Daphne Bartrum.

March 1977

CHAPTER I: DISCONTINUATION: A NEGLECTED TOPIC?

Discontinuation of contraceptive practice is a complex social, cultural, psychological and often medical problem involving numerous contraceptive methods and channels, and characterized by a range of variables often independent of family planning programmes. It is a component of several patterns of contraceptive use and is as yet only partially understood. The problem of programme discontinuation is first the difficulty of identifying the patterns to which so-called 'drop-outs' belong and second of developing responses for specific patterns. This chapter describes the rather oblique way in which the issue of programme and method discontinuation has come to be defined.

There are very few papers explicitly on discontinuation, but quite a number which shed light more or less directly upon it. These are largely demographic and biomedical, providing necessary but incomplete information as part of knowledge, attitude and practice (KAP) studies, clinical and field trials of new contraceptive methods, or programme records and follow-ups.

The first problem is to discover how and why the literature has grown in this way. We need to understand the nature and influence of current concepts of discontinuation before we can begin to explore other ideas and methods which may increase our understanding.

1 A Short History of 'Drop-outs'

There is no critical bibliography and assessment of materials related to family planning drop-outs. This is probably because discontinuation was overshadowed in the first flush of success in family planning. Tabulation and comparison of initial 'acceptors' was and still is a dramatic way of recording this success and of justifying greater programme expenditure. Consequently programme discontinuation has been approached on the whole through studies primarily directed to counting positive aspects.

Early questions about contraceptive use and disuse were addressed to family planning 'practice'. KAP studies, even after hundreds of surveys were completed, were usually addressed to 'ever' use, and if so, to 'which method', 'how recently', and to current or potential 'satisfaction'.[1]

The main purpose of these data was to make the case for family planning programmes; beyond establishing a generalized need, little was or could be done with it. As Cleland recently noted[2], these studies attend primarily to demographic categories and have little explanatory power, whereas the need is for information about what people actually do in specific local situations.

One curious characteristic of KAP studies has been the distinction between questions about practice on the one hand and attitudes on the other, as if they could be neatly separated. The issue of continuation-discontinuation strikes precisely at this point, for the process by which users adopt, change or stop using a method (or methods or various services) is a complex and evolving set of actions. Neither demographic categories nor sweeping distinctions of 'practices' and 'attitudes' cope with this. It was quickly realized (140, 243, 245, 347) that 'acceptance' and 'practice' were meaningless unless as part of consistent patterns of continuation. The idea that patterns of continuation also imply patterns of discontinuation has waited much longer to receive attention.

---

1 The Population Council. A Manual for Surveys of Fertility and Family Planning: Knowledge, Attitudes Practices. New York, 1970.

2 Cleland, J. 'A Critique of KAP Studies and Some Suggestions for Their Improvement' Studies in Family Planning, 4, 2, 42-47, 1973.

The KAP approach has influenced the study of continuation and discontinuation. The study and presentation of materials on continuation have been treated in the same way as data on acceptance. Calculations of discontinuation rates, because apparently precise and scientific, have often seemed a sufficient end in themselves. Basic demographic and socio-economic characteristics (by acceptance or period of use) have been reported, almost completely shorn of their social context.

Categories tabulated and compared for the purpose of demonstrating certain programme needs and effects may not be the most suitable to exploring contraceptive practice. Different terminologies and methods are needed for different ends. Without doubt the most influential approach to the study of contraceptive use has been that developed to assess the 'use-effectiveness' of specific contraceptive methods. This has supplemented demographic and attitudinal surveys with clinical questions.

Questions about 'length of use' appear, for example, in Kenny's early reports on the family planning programmes in Korea and Taiwan, and in some of the pilot projects in these areas (12, 54, 56, 137). From the first, questions about continuation and discontinuation were wrapped up in the histories of particular programmes, national and international, as shown in the first Taiwan IUD follow-up report (245):

> "... to measure adequately the effectiveness of the IUD among acceptors, it is not enough to calculate merely a pregnancy rate among wearers. It is essential to know the proportion wearing the device at specified intervals after insertion and for those not still wearing it, the time and circumstance of device loss. Then too, retention of the IUD may vary among different segments of a population. For purposes of allocating effort where it will count most in a large-scale family planning programme, it is imperative to know

whether such differentials exist. A deeper and more useful understanding of the use-effectiveness of the IUD in a particular population is gained by investigating the manner in which pregnancy, expulsion, and removal rates vary among wearers of differing demographic and social characteristics."

This statement encapsulates the major concerns of research on continuation and discontinuation at the time (February, 1967) and ever since. These are: the question of how intervals are to be specified; the selection of variables for monitoring circumstances by socio-demographic categories; and the classification of reasons for discontinuation by pregnancy, expulsion and removal.

As we shall see in Chapter II, the desire to keep these simple classifications regardless of social and cultural variations has resulted in ambiguous data. Looking back to the 1960's and 1970's when use-effectiveness techniques were used, it is as if researchers had assumed that clinical effectiveness was the primary or even the only factor in contraceptive use, without regard to the social and cultural aspects of discontinuation. This unbalanced situation has shaped the entire course of discontinuation studies.

The manner in which discontinuation is now discussed owes a great deal to the development of the IUD. While the first generation devices, notably loops, were being made the basis of early programmes in Taiwan and Korea, and later of the International Post-partum Programme (I.P.P.) (306, 385), and while research was beginning on the 'second generation' of devices, writers such as Tietze and Potter applied life table techniques to the measurement of use-effectiveness. A substantial portion of this methodology was carried out under the IUD Co-operative Statistical Programme (C.S.P.) (338, 341, 343, 347). The way in which we assess contraceptive use is still to a large extent moulded by the prospect held out by the IUD in the early days of a single device of long-term effectiveness making few demands on the day to day motivation of either user or programme. We are much better at monitoring the success, failure and probable causes of single-method events than we are of the use of several methods of varying effectiveness available from a variety of sources.

The IUD was a seemingly ideal contraceptive with high use-effectiveness. There were clear-cut criteria for the presence or absence of the device, immediately indicating use or discontinuation, and efficacy or risk. It lent itself to measurement in a way that no other contraceptive could. IUD users depended more upon medical services for insertion and removal than oral contraceptive or 'traditional' method users. Acceptances were comparatively easy to record and discontinuation rates could be computed by the life table technique.

Furthermore the IUD seemed to suggest a way around the complicated social, cultural and psychological factors involved in trying to increase use. We can imagine a simplified argument on this score to run as follows: The motivational question, notably the complete absence of a necessary link between attitudes and practices, is an especially difficult one. In fact, it is more often than not beyond us. Not only are values and motivations subtle and changeable but the difficulty of understanding any expression of them may require a good knowledge of local language and idiom. The methods most suited to providing programmatic information (surveys and record-keeping systems), are the least suited to what becomes, ipso facto, unprogrammatic information[3], i.e. data needed to understand

---

3 However, some important efforts have been made to improve the quality of programmatic data. See: Caldwell, J.C., The Study of Fertility and Fertility Change in Tropical Africa. World Fertility Survey Occasional Papers, No. 7., 1974.

reactions to the programme but not confined to programme service statistics.

However, if a particular method (i.e. the IUD) lessens the motivational components and if the principal objective of study in any case is duration of use, then the tenuous connection of dispositions and actions may for the moment be set aside. Attention may instead be concentrated upon identifying favourable factors and upon keeping medical complications to a minimum. Although demographic factors such as age, education and parity are not explanatory, they may identify the problem clearly enough. For example, parity data suggest the points at which women really begin to think in terms of limiting their families. Medical reasons for termination by demographic category may suggest improvements in devices or in the programme itself for specific types of users.

This line of argument would suggest that the potential of the IUD lay in side-stepping fundamental and apparently intractable problems - a research priority much the same as that of KAP surveys.

IUD-dominated programmes have given way to programmes offering several methods (253). None of these methods or combinations lends itself so readily to assessment. The frequency and extent of use of oral contraceptives and so-called 'traditional methods' - condoms, foam, rhythm, diaphragm and jelly - are difficult to determine. More or less arbitrary starting and cut-off points are necessary (48) if method use is to be analysed as for the IUD. The influence of sterilization and particularly of abortion should be included. Thus the accumulation of multiple starts and stops with several methods of different effectiveness, and with multiple and possibly unidentified sources of supply, makes up a statistical puzzle now recognized as beyond the scope of current measurement techniques. (49, 255, and below Chapter II, section 1: Methods of Measurement).

The recent multi-method period has also seen a considerable expansion of social, psychological and even of anthropological studies directed to problems of discontinuation: husband-wife communication, commercial distribution, the value of children, insertion of contraceptives by para-medical personnel, and others. Only recently however has discontinuation been linked directly to ongoing social processes. Examples include projects such as Korean Mothers' Clubs (382), special follow-ups to re-assure new users (13-16, 46), or the postpartum and post-abortion family planning programmes (17, 40, 71, 78, 88, 115, 143, 271, 305, 306, 371, 375, 376, 385), which try to adapt programmes to local cultural patterns. They use existing networks for economic development or maternal and child care, or, in the case of special follow-ups, attempt to get as many women as possible to follow the example of older women who have completed their families.

Despite increased attention to social factors, the inappropriateness of existing measurements for methods other than the IUD or for everyday contexts of contraceptive use, and the disturbingly high drop-out rates, discontinuation has not become a priority area of study. On the whole, reporting of discontinuation tends to follow the older medical-directed priorities, perhaps with somewhat more elaborate categories. This type of study predominates even in the more recent literature (7, 9, 40, 51, 147, 151, 214, 268, 287, 309, 322, 361).

2 How Past Definitions Limit Current Understanding

A number of reasons may be cited for this seeming neglect, including limits to available information, the very success of use-effectiveness evaluations and a certain negativism which surrounds the topic of drop-outs.

(a) Many articles (1, 167, 183, 197, 201, 207, 275, 282, 287, 306, 309) report only standard information about use and discontinuation because that is the only information available from studies based on clinic records and follow-ups, or comparative trials of new methods.

(b) Life table methods for the IUD are elegant and imitable; their validity for clinical trials of new methods is established; they have been widely used and reported (49, 243, 246, 303, 338, 340, 345, 347, 353, 354 etc.). There is a natural tendency to carry out well planned and executed programmes in an already established field and to measure that which lends itself to measurement. Evaluations of condom continuation (131, 150, 225, 333) rhythm (176, 342, 335) or of vaginal contraceptives (24, 48, 52, 72, 339, 374), for example, are much fewer. Success in the description of certain methods may not only divert attention from others, but keep research focused on methods rather than users (140).

(c) The complexity, multiplicity and lack of precision characteristic of patterns of use and discontinuation outstrip the capacity of the life table while the statistical or computerized methods ultimately required are too abstract to be widely used. But there is a more pressing problem: lack of adequate data, and indecision as to what data would really be useful. How great a proportion of discontinuers return to contraception and for what reason? When do they return? Are there patterns of discontinuation and return to contraception? Of those apparently lost to family planning how many have discontinued because of age, sterility, mortality, divorce, separation, migration or unresolvable medical problems? Are the remaining drop-outs who could return to contraceptive use if encouraged worth the effort and cost? Lack of information about these groups contributes to the attitude, noted by Cernada, that the drop-out problem is 'better ignored' (44).

(d) A last consideration is the moral connotation of the word "discontinuer". The contrast between terms used for discontinuation - 'drop-outs, 'attrition', 'deserters', 'failures', 'terminators', 'defectors', 'defaulters', 'quitters', 'enders', 'resisters' - and those associated with continuation - 'acceptors', 'patients', 'clients' - suggests that any further look at discontinuation is an exercise in fault-finding. It seems that either the user or the programme must be blamed. Discontinuation then becomes a sensitive topic. Positive or promising performance is more generally written up than programme disappointments. A central issue in the approach to discontinuation must be to eliminate this implicit negativism. Either discontinuation is a serious programme problem which must be given priority; or it will have to be resolved into a set of apparently more fruitful questions best approached in other ways.

Each of these factors - lack of appropriate information, the limitations of available measures, method rather than user-orientation, and the sensitivity of evaluation - are important in understanding recent literature on clinic discontinuation, (35, 36, 68, 94, 97, 141, 142, 144, 205, 208, 218, 219, 220, 261, 292, 294, 301, 319, 320, 362). Some studies are modelled closely on use-effectiveness studies (141, 309, 360). A number (35, 208, 219, 261, 292, 301) suggest that they are modelled in <u>reaction</u> to method-orientated studies: they all but ignore the substantial role medical problems play in discontinuation. Others are directed to specific topics such as waiting times, distance factors and insertions by paramedical personnel (82, 144, 269, 270, 386). This type of study redresses the balance by showing the potential influence of programme operations on discontinuation, but method and operational aspects of discontinuation are still viewed separately. In this way available writings on discontinuation exert a strong influence on any attempt to examine the problem differently.

Systematic studies of use-effectiveness, or of attitudes about contraception are achieved by strictly limiting the object of attention. A research tradition is defined not only by the characteristic questions it asks, but by the systematic exclusion of other questions. It is often difficult to foresee the effects of this isolation; once particular research techniques and the characteristic descriptions they produce are accepted, these descriptions become identified with the problem or issue. In this example, those who stop using a contraceptive or who stop coming into a clinic are labelled 'drop-outs'; this leads to rather loaded questions as to why the person 'dropped-out'. Similarly classification of unfavourable 'attitudes' or irregular 'practice' encourages the view that these people are 'resisters' or that the problem lies in a 'gap' between knowledge, attitudes and practices. The likelihood that these are adaptive responses to a local situation can be pointed out, but not systematically considered by these research techniques. In short, the success of a particular mode of description results in that description passing for reality. Further, there is a definite suggestion that other aspects of a problem, in order to be properly and scientifically considered, must first receive a similar 'rigorous' formulation.

The problem is that not all social phenomena may be treated in the same way; there are different sorts of 'rigorous' formulation. A fundamental and open question is whether existing research techniques accurately translate relevant aspects of other cultures with very different structures and patterns of action. As long as existing research techniques are maintained, the unbalanced state of our knowledge cannot be righted by adding cultural questions or by employing local personnel. Some new approach to the problem will be necessary.

The development of use-effectiveness research shows how an excellent research technique which resolved a particular and difficult problem (how to assess clinical effectiveness) comes to monopolize the evaluation of everyday contexts of use. By its exclusions it points the way to other questions and methods which need to be developed. It also underlines the danger of importing even proven methodologies into apparently related topic areas without first considering the individuality of the new area of study.

CHAPTER II: MEASURING DISCONTINUATION

The last chapter showed a tension between programmatic and unprogrammatic information - that is, between data needed for operations and easily collected, and data which seem unsuited to collection and are of varying relevance. The first variety consists mostly of socio-demographic and medical categories, supplemented by a few attitudinal queries ('limiters' versus 'spacers'; son preferences; etc.). The second may include everything from ideas about menstruation and bleeding, to clinic structure, to the state of the economy. The main issue unanswered by medical and socio-demographic studies of contraceptive use continues to be the usefulness of research for programme resource allocation. The main question is whether patterns of use and disuse if better understood, could become a guide through the maze of possible influences on drop-out rates.

This section gives an answer to the question: How far will existing 'programmatic' data resolve questions about drop-outs? Despite the generally low comparability of studies, an outline for action begins to emerge. A review of life table techniques shows that they do not at present help in following multiple patterns of use; however, they do indicate broad trends in the age and parity of users which suggests that there are older women of higher parity who have fairly clear ideas about whether they want further children, and a generally younger group of women of lower parity who show considerable ambivalence. Further socio-demographic information on education, residence, income, and so on, does not account for either the differences between these two loosely defined groups, or the often considerable variations within them. The age and parity pattern is too general to be of use as an audience segmentation strategy for resource allocation.

Use-effectiveness studies also indicate consistently high patterns of early discontinuation of oral contraception due to side effects, although the inter-relation of medical, cultural, social and psychological factors in this is not clear. A similar situation exists regarding medical and personal reasons for IUD removal. Studies generally do not attempt to identify patterns of discontinuation and subsequent use in these categories. What happens after termination is the subject of Chapter 3.

1 *Methods of Measurement*

Measures of contraceptive use, effects and side-effects were first important in a clinical context in which contraceptives were special medical techniques. The development of measures has followed the pattern laid down by biomathematics and demography, based on the life table. The first application of the life table method to fertility control is recorded by Potter (243, 244, 249). As noted in Chapter 1 the method is particularly suited to the IUD, and was described in a considerable number of studies, articles, summaries and manuals (49, 303, 338, 347, 353). Comment here is confined to some points in the logic of the method which limit its usefulness for the study of discontinuation.

The life table is a method of determining rates among events which occur over different periods of time. It includes in a single model a large number of individual variations, including the number and timing of events, differences among individual users, and defects in available information. Information is inevitably partial because variations in dates of entry into a programme give data on different lengths of use and different stages of use. A certain number of users are lost to follow-up or continue beyond the cut off point of a study, so that their contraceptive histories are incomplete.

The life table cannot account for each of these variations but schedules them all in the same way on the basis of risk:

> "Perhaps the largest source of variation, however, is the unequal regularity with which contraception is practiced. In the same sample an intermittent practice of contraception by some couples may mean monthly risks of conception many times higher than those of other couples who are wholly regular in their precautions. Naturally the high-risk women conceive more rapidly than the low risk women and as a consequence, during a given pregnancy interval the composition of the sample, in terms of who remains at risk, is continually changing. For this reason the experience of a group of contraceptors is advantageously viewed as a process changing through exposure time. As successive months of exposure elapse, the accident-prone are selectively removed by pregnancy to leave behind a more and more homogeneously low-risk remainder."(244)

In effect, exposure to risk is held constant and the table records the proportion of a fertile population which successfully 'survives' each month without pregnancy or other cause for discontinuation. The various causes may be tabulated independently as net termination rates; the total is then additive of the component kinds of discontinuation.

Tables I and II list cumulative rates in a number of studies for the IUD and oral contraceptives respectively, and Tables III and IV give respective breakdowns by termination status. As Tables I and II suggest, rates of discontinuation are consistently high. For the IUD, discontinuation is near one-third in the first year, and near one-half by the end of the second. Pill discontinuation is higher still, approaching one-half at the end of one year, and two-thirds by the second. These figures, though subject to variations in field conditions, reporting and in methods of study (see below) suggest sizeable dissatisfaction with methods, even when some users make several attempts.

Unfortunately, the user who tries again, with or without the same method, cannot be followed by the life table technique. The 'multiple decrement' life table just described accommodates the user who restarts the same method by treating her as a new case. The rates listed in Tables I - IV are mostly 'first method' rates, including restarts; 'first segment' rates record only users' first continuous stretch of contraception with a single method. The extent and sequence of restarts and reinsertions is not regularly reported.

Data on shifts to alternative methods are not consistently reported (cf. Tables III and IV), and existing accounts are limited both by the relatively short periods to which they refer and by the influence of unmonitored contraception from other sources. Nevertheless the extent of discontinuation suggests that the impact of programmes viewed demographically or otherwise, depends on a combination of methods.

An adaptation of the life table method, under the term 'extended use-effectiveness' (341) does provide an all-method accounting, but precludes information on the continuity and breaks-in-use of several methods. Instead, the interval is taken as the entire period between a given starting point (e.g. first use of a particular method) and the next conception, cut-off date, lack of need, or loss to follow-up, whichever comes first. Tietze and Lewit (341) in an exposition of the concept note that

> "... periods of non-use, with or without exposure to the risk of pregnancy that last one month or longer and are followed by resumption of use are omitted; periods of use that precede and follow these

> interruptions are added; and the duration is treated as a single continuing period."

They also note that this approach is suitable to overall programme evaluation, but its limits are well noted by Potter and Avery (255):

> "Another strength of the extended use-effectiveness approach is that it transcends the complexity of method shifts and interruptions of contraceptive use, thereby retrieving simplicity and feasibility of analysis. This strength is also its weakness. By transcending complexity, it sacrifices detail and wastes information. One learns nothing directly about the acceptability and use-effectiveness of the contraceptives that produce the derived distribution of intervals to the next conception (or live birth)."

In the same article, Avery suggests the application of some more sophisticated mathematical processes to the problem, but his exploration is admittedly tentative.

This is the current state of the measurement apparatus available for monitoring intervals of use and discontinuation. Two implications follow from this. One is that there is no available 'easy way out' which, in the manner of KAP surveys or use-effectiveness studies sets aside socio-cultural factors in favour of relatively simple measures. The life table method makes systematic use of varying and often deficient data, but it excludes aspects of contraceptive use - sequences of use and discontinuation, often involving more than one method - which are essential to understanding discontinuation. The method of analysis discourages the construction of a more adequate data base. The second implication, to which we now turn, is that interpreting discontinuation without regard to local influences must be in important respects misleading. Information collected in the use-effectiveness format can give only very general guidance to programme efforts.

The major problem in using life table data lies in the stereotyped 'reasons for termination'. The accumulation of net rates by reason is of interest only if the reasons themselves are valid. The varieties of termination usually studied are a basic set devised for medical purposes, but undeveloped with reference to social, cultural and psychological factors. The Co-operative Statistical Program for the Evaluation of IUDs (C.S.P.) (338, 341, 347), identified the main categories, which may be summarized:

A. Accidental pregnancy: Includes all conceptions in the period with the IUD in place, or as long as the wearer believes it to be in place, i.e., including unnoticed expulsions. (Some expulsions thus are classified as pregnancies).

B. Expulsion: Includes wearer noticed expulsions, and removals of partial expulsions from the cervix. (Some removals thus are classified as expulsions).

C. Removal for bleeding and/or pain: Includes cases in which bleeding/pain are attributed to the IUD either by the wearer or the investigator.

D. Removal for other medical reasons: Includes removals because of physical complaints by the wife or husband attributed to the IUD, whether considered relevant by the investigator or not; also includes removals for treatment of intercurrent conditions, even if apparently unrelated to the device.

E. Removal for planning a pregnancy.

F. Removal for other personal reasons: Includes removals for non-medical reasons, but excludes cases where no reason is given, where contraception is no longer needed, and removals at the investigators choice.

G. Loss to follow-up: Includes women three or more months overdue for a scheduled appointment, and for whom no information could be gained by follow-up.

In this classification the overlap of 'expulsion', 'removal' and 'accidental pregnancy' may or may not be significant, but it reminds us that even physical events are not simple to classify. Since the categories generally used for oral contraceptives - 'pregnancy' (accidental or not), 'side-effects and medical reasons', 'personal' reasons, 'other' and 'loss to follow-up' - are similar, the following remarks apply to them as well in considering both the reliability of information provided by this scheme, and the extent to which it gives a realistic picture of how discontinuation happens.

The classification appears to give equal status to users' and investigators' statements. But the equal status is only an appearance, for it is the investigator who writes down what has happened. Both user and investigator will prefer certain kinds of reports and relevant background information may be excluded, consciously or not, from the interview. Several other forces are at work in shaping the data:

(a) The classification rests on a separation of medical and non-medical reasons. This overlaps to an undetermined extent an implicit distinction between physical and non-physical (personal, social, cultural, etc.) reasons. An important question regarding drop-outs is whether, with a little more support, they might put up with physical discomforts. It is impossible to identify such a group under the classification, and general attempts at reassurance for all new users have been shown to be unproductive and costly (46). To take another example, considerable emphasis has been laid recently on social and cultural variations in the amount of irregular bleeding or pain a woman is willing to endure (120). The traditional medical classification in terms of the 'menstrual cycle' has been thoroughly revised [4]. Medical/non medical distinctions make for unanswerable questions along the lines of 'Is it really medical or is it personal or psychological?'

(b) The classification in effect ignores the way in which people learn to express bodily experiences and develop skills for coping with them, even though the impetus behind population programmes has been to teach, indoctrinate, or identify relevant indigenous beliefs and skills called 'family planning'. Several writers have noticed that users <u>are</u> developing skills for coping with clinics: they learn to provide complaints and reasons recognized in the classificatory scheme, which means they are saved the trouble or embarrassment of explaining their discontinuation. (45, 233).

(c) The unreliability of post hoc statements about family size or unwanted pregnancies is well

---

4 Rodriguez, G., Faundes-Latham, A.. Atkinson, L.E. An Approach to the Analysis of Menstrual Patterns in the Critical Evaluation of Contraceptives. Studies in Family Planning, 7, 2, 42-51, 1976.

known. The same is true for statements about the regularity of contraceptive practice (119). The difficulty of separating the 'intentionally' from the 'accidentally' pregnant has been noted (132), and this probably applies to some women who 'have not noticed' expulsions, or who are caught up in incomplete patterns of pill use (57).

(d) The classification is very rationalistic, since all disconnections are given the status of 'reasons'. These include religious beliefs, rumours, folk explanations of various kinds, patterns of avoidance, and correct and incorrect scientific diagnoses. Not all of these carry the same weight, and a given user may have several and inter-related 'reasons' for continuation.

(e) A number of important factors, notably the accessibility and extent of change to alternative methods, are not regularly reported. Finally, the classification is not always strictly adhered.

The purpose of this somewhat detailed comment on the C.S.P. classification is to suggest that inattention to socio-cultural and psychological factors reduces the credibility of cut-and-dried medical typologies. We can easily imagine how cultural reasons related to bleeding, for example, may lie behind the discontinuation of a group of women who would be indistinguishable by medical/non-medical classifications. Cultural and psychological factors seem particularly unlikely to receive direct expression: they are not so much 'reasons' as assumptions having to do with a whole way of life.

An individual case involving irregular bleeding, complaints about side-effects, and perhaps a medical history including attempts with several methods, could conceivably be classified in several ways. The 'other personal' category (F.) which would be appropriate for cultural bleeding factors, is by no means the most obvious. The natural tendency for a doctor might be to record medical indications, as Tietze and Lewit note in their Ninth Report (343):

> "The distinction between medical and personal reasons for removal was not always unequivocal; doubtful cases were classified as medical."

The finding that medical complications predominate reasons for discontinuing the IUD and pill (275), must be read with the medical orientation of these studies in mind. Where there is some uncertainty, but a clear desire for removal or stoppage on the part of the user, classifications (C), (D) and (F) all become possible. Through frustration or subterfuge, the user might also find her way into categories (E) and (G), and eventually even (A). There are no studies to throw light on recording and classification procedures.

The main question is whether all the important factors in discontinuation are being brought out by this approach which has provided most of the available information on discontinuation and now provides the conventional baseline for further study.

The materials recorded in Tables I-IV come from rather different types of study. The majority are based on a combination of clinic records and follow-up surveys. Several sources of bias in these methods and materials may be noted. Studies which record differences in the quality of the two types of source invariably cite the unreliability of records (1, 7, 183, 211). This typically takes the form of under-reporting of discontinuation, and occasionally of fabricating figures for contraceptive practice. There is thus some reason to doubt studies based upon clinic records alone (32, 147, 167, 279, 282, 309). On the other hand, checks on the representativeness of samples do not necessarily ensure their reliability. Frequently there is merely random selection from clinic records (1, 7, 45, 141, 183, 216, 315, 322, 350). However, insofar as users and discontinuers make up two different self-selected portions of the target population, this method may only accomplish randomization out of an unrandom sample. For example, almost all studies report a sizeable loss to follow-up due to inaccurate reporting of user's addresses; this factor seems highly unlikely to be random.

Controlled studies are rare (15, 46, 109, 270, 382); even the ability to control for certain factors within a particular social and cultural setting does not ensure comparability with other settings. Reasonably reliable national demographic data may provide a standard against which to judge sample bias in particular areas.

The uniformity of the C.S.P. is no doubt responsible for whatever comparability these studies have. But it is difficult to know whether the practice behind this reporting format is at all similar. Moreover, information on the conduct and analysis of surveys is not always reported, notably (i) the period of the survey; (ii) the nature of the loss to follow-up; (iii) the mode of calculation of rates; (iv) background information on the locations studied; (v) definitions of 'discontinuation' or 'dropping-out'; (vi) the type of the staff conducting the interview; and (vii) special circumstances of a study.

Use of the term 'discontinuation' requires definition. Obviously the extent of drop-out increases as criteria of acceptance relax. A number of studies report small numbers of pill 'acceptors' who never take a single pill (80,130,138,366), but this has only in one instance been followed up (293). All reports on the first months of pill and IUD usage, with very occasional exception, show the highest user loss in this period, a loss consistently attributed to medically related reasons. There is little cause to doubt this finding, and no question that it represents a significant portion of those ready and willing to practise contraception. These are individuals who _have_ tried the methods and _stopped_, which is what 'acceptance' and 'dropping out' come down to. The conditions of initial use are one of the main mysteries of the problem of discontinuation. This part of the problem lacks definition.

Part of the problem is procedural: at what point should the cut-off be placed for measurement purposes? For the IUD, expulsion or removal without reinsertion or method change is identifiable: the device is not _in situ_ at the recording date. For the oral and traditional methods there is usually some arbitrary point of last contact which may be used as a standard. The C.S.P. adopted a three-month period following a missed check-up. Studies vary as to whether they assume a woman is a continuing user until she has finished all the pills she has been given, or only some of them. Others may stipulate some period since last contact. The term discontinuation thus lacks standardization.

The organizational contexts of these studies are very different. Some present the findings of hospital outpatient services, characteristically with a small, self-selected intake over a long period (20, 32, 207, 279, 309, 315, 359). Some report on similar services within larger specialized projects (27, 40, 78, 88, 121, 143, 239, 271, 306, 385), others are connected with special education, communications or other projects having to do with family planning clinics in national programmes (7, 13, 14, 15, 46, 87, 132, 168, 220, 233, 269, 322, 359, 380). Finally, data from the C.S.P. more or less set the pace for other and later research on contraceptive use. It is interesting to note the limitation placed by the authors on their material:

> "... the usefulness of the information provided by the C.S.P. based on experience with IUDs among clinic populations in the United States, is diminishing since it is not generally applicable to conditions in other countries ... Furthermore, the clinics co-operating in the CSP were, for the most part, strongly research oriented, and not only provided better medical care but also took a greater interest in the individual women than is usually possible in a health setting." (343)

On the whole it is difficult to distinguish special influences due to the various types of study. Many are the first services and research of their kind in a given area and this suggests that subsequent events may be different. The course and effects of a programme 'settling in' are not well understood. In the next section we will turn to the general findings of this body of research. They show that contrary to Tietze and Lewit's comment on the limitations of the C.S.P., several of the aspects of continuation and discontinuation it identified appear to hold more widely. However, the shortcomings of this approach noted above suggest that this similarity is unreliable due to the limited scope of the research methods used.

2 *Summary of Findings*

The findings can be summarized in the following six points:

(a) First method discontinuation rates for all reasons as indicated in Tables I-II are initially high but gradually decline. A substantial portion - up to one-half in some cases (74, 130, 201) - drop out in the first 3 to 6 months. Ross et.al. in an earlier synopsis (275), placed IUD discontinuation at 23 to 38 per 100 users per first year, and 44 to 51 at two years. Corresponding rates for oral contraceptive discontinuation were between 38% and 45% at one year. These figures hold up fairly well four years later. It is now possible to add pill discontinuation rates at two years, averaging about 75%.

(b) When subdivided by 'reasons' (Table III) IUD discontinuation occurs primarily by removal for bleeding or pain and related medical-physical categories; expulsion is the second most frequent reason. One third of pill discontinuation (Table IV) is attributed to medical and side-effects, followed by approximately one-fourth of the reasons listed as 'personal'. Pregnancy and planned pregnancy are the next most frequently cited events for both methods. Physical-related reasons seem the most consistently cited.

(c) The length of continuous use needed to attain desired contraceptive effect varies, of course, among individuals, even if the initial average age is higher (for example, over age thirty - 90, 132, 147, 169, 172, 188, 322, 350, 380), it is easy to see that for many women both limitation and spacing will require periods of use of more than two years. Sizeable numbers of women are evidently not achieving this with their first method. Data for three or more years are not regularly available. What <u>is</u> available indicates that by the third year IUD discontinuation rates approach two-thirds of the initial users, including reinsertions. The downward trend then continues and tapers slightly. There are few reports available on longer periods of use of oral contraceptives.

(d) Both IUD and pill show consistently better continuation as age and parity increase. Most users are 25 to 34; parity and number of living children are reported interchangeably, and 'higher' numbers are reported variously as 3 - 4 - 5 - or more births. Studies indicating this or similar broad patterns of acceptance are listed below.

IUD: 1, 7, 8, 12, 17, 51, 61, 90, 106, 167, 172, 183, 233, 245, 287, 306, 322, 382.

Oral: 7, 31, 32, 45, 50, 132, 172, 183, 188, 207, 211, 282, 306, 361, 379, 380.

Some studies note that this pattern declines in the 'over-35' and 'more than 5 births' categories (45, 306, 361).

Ross et. al. (275) compare acceptance patterns suggesting that pill acceptors represent on the whole a younger element within the 25-34 age group. Taiwan studies (61, 90, 107), and writings on postpartum family planning (88) confirm a younger age pattern for continuation, suggesting use of the IUD for birth limitation and oral contraception for spacing. The inference is that spacing is a less strongly motivated family planning strategy, which accords with the higher pregnancy and discontinuation rates characteristic of younger women. American studies (276, 278) indicate that younger 'spacers' are more likely to fail to prevent conception. The pill is responsible for a sizeable portion of this failure (though a main force behind the overall decline in unwanted fertility in the U.S. in the last ten years). There seems to be some general agreement on this combination of demographic (age and parity), attitudinal (limiting or spacing) and method (pill or IUD) variables, although it has not been confirmed more widely. The implication for discontinuation studies is strategic, suggesting two target audiences: one somewhat older with fairly definite family planning goals, and one somewhat younger with more ambivalent feelings. However, it seems unlikely that this strategy would work so simply. Age and number of children do not altogether account for differentials in oral and IUD performance. Sivin (249) shows low oral continuation rates in all subgroups by age and number of children, even including stated desire for children. Avery (8) notes that after two years IUD discontinuation cannot be differentiated by these characteristics. The limiting/spacing dichotomy in effect assumes single-minded motivations on the part of the user: while this makes some sense for so-called 'limiters', the case is not so simple for others. Finally, use of other methods, and gaps in use, are not accounted for.

An alternative is suggested by Liu, Chow and Abbey (194) and substantiated by studies in Taiwan (8, 51, 214) viz: two patterns involving those who are and those who are not likely to continue with the IUD for an extended period. A high risk group characteristically drops out in the first six months, with a subsequent gradual decline in the probability of discontinuation which approaches a constant and low level. In the first two years, young women of low parity and higher education are more likely to discontinue. After two years, discontinuation rates decline substantially for all users, effectively eliminating differentials for all groups. The number of reinsertions after three years is only slightly less than the number of discontinuations, suggesting that by this time continuing users consider the IUD a more or less permanent method.

This work has two important features. First, it is based on actual events for a lengthy period (six to nine years). Second, it does not depend on inferred values and motivations. Since re-insertion and continuation figures usually exclude removals, the method identifies this latter group as a key drop-out population. The disadvantage of the Taiwanese studies for comparative purposes is the singularity of the programme, especially its emphasis on the IUD. Moots and Chang (214) argue that programme effectiveness depends on quick response to discontinuation and they note a lower level but consistent use of condoms, diaphragm and jelly, rhythm, pills, and sterilizations tending to stabilize at two to three years after first insertion. The importance of gaps in use following first terminations is clear for all methods and programmes; but the patterns of subsequent use of alternative methods where there is no emphasis on reinsertions are not so well defined.

(e) The importance of longitudinal data of this kind is corroborated by the finding that once longer patterns of continuation are laid down, they are sustained: the longer a user continues with

a chosen method, the longer she is likely to go on with it (50, 51, 61, 74, 100). Moreover, it has been noted that continuers as a group tend to have higher fecundability (123); hence the importance of continuing with some method, even if not the first. Both of these points take on added significance with the finding that younger women of lower parity form an increasing proportion of initial users (61, 90, 153, 254, 379). Postpartum family planning programmes have shown that significant patterns of continuation can be established for younger women of lower parity, with continuation over increasingly long periods (88, 306).
It is not permissible to infer from this a heightened interest in family planning or spacing by younger groups; such trends may be only a consequence of prior acceptance patterns in which older groups predominated (254). Understanding rather than postulating patterns of use in these groups becomes increasingly important.

(f) Many studies of contraceptive use include an education variable, usually on the basis of level reached (illiterate, primary, secondary, further). A negative relationship with length of use is frequently indicated, most users having completed or partially completed primary education, but in which illiterate users may be a significant group (1, 8, 12, 17, 45, 51, 90, 107, 169, 172, 188, 211, 322). A number of authors (7, 45, 132) point out that this pattern seems to be a function of age. Older groups as a rule have less education and seem more likely to fall into incomplete-primary or illiterate categories. Completed primary education (which represents a higher educational level in many areas) relates to the increasing trends in slightly younger initial users. Finally, a number of studies record education as making no difference (45, 183, 349, 352, 371). Other study variables include: income, occupation (husband or wife), prior contraceptive experience, prior abortion experience, duration of marriage, nuclear versus extended family, and urban-rural differences. Compilations of findings from IUD surveys (167), more general assessments (275), and attempts to assess income[5] and abortion (348) in related surveys, express dissatisfaction with the completeness, comparability and reliability of the information.

If we compare these broad findings with those reported for the C.S.P. (343), several points emerge in common. These are the conclusions of the C.S.P. :

(i) removals account for most closures, even when removals for planned pregnancy are excluded;

(ii) removals for bleeding or pain are highest in younger women of low parity, and decline with increases in age and parity;

(iii) removal risk is highest in the first year, and then declines gradually;

(iv) expulsion risk is highest in the first year, and then drops more steeply to low levels;

(v) pregnancy risk is highest in the first year, and then is somewhat less.

Probably the most significant difference is the finding that the fraction, roughly 3/5 of users, continuing

---

5 MacDonald, M., Mueller, E. The Measurement of Income in Fertility Surveys. Taiwan Population Studies Centre Working Paper No. 24. 1973.

beyond two years in the C.S.P. falls to nearly 1/2 for the IUD and 1/4 for the pill. This confirms other reports (275) that IUD and pill discontinuation is higher in mass programmes than in clinical trials.

The consistency of basic medical and demographic findings is less an argument for the comparability of these studies, than it is for the obviousness of the facts available to this approach. As Chen, Su and Chow (51) note in their study of reinsertion, it is reasonable to expect these patterns to hold for later segments of use:

> "Past analyses of the retention rates of the first segment of IUD use of various programs indicate that, although the values of some parameters may differ from one program to another, the general principles governing IUD retention and correlates of retention with various sociological and medical variables appear to be the same for the majority of programs studied. It is assumed, therefore, that the basic principles governing the reinsertion behaviour of IUD users outlined in this article will apply to similar programs in other parts of the world."

What, then, are the programmatic implications of these measures?

The following interpretation is suggested.

(a) Physical complications are a given feature of the two main modern contraceptive methods, and a significant number of women will not be able to use them continuously at least at first.

(b) The extent of personal, cultural, social and psychological factors in this pattern of initial difficulty and the extent to which they can be manipulated to improve continuation is unknown.

The emphasis must shift from monitoring method effects to understanding patterns of use and discontinuation.

(c) The key to assessing quality of services and programme effectiveness lies in understanding how people act after dropping a method. Appropriate allocation of programme resources depends on the pattern of: restarts, method changes, abortion, substitution of method sources, unprotected discontinuation and loss to follow-up.

(d) These events make up a longitudinal set of patterns, in which users will probably occupy several categories over time. Record keeping systems will need to be oriented to this task, and new measurement techniques devised. There are several developments in this direction already (74, 79, 94, 102, 194).

(e) Tabulation and correlation of age, parity and other socio-demographic variables with simplified reasons for discontinuation at best suggest that a large percentage of women of reproductive age are not being assimilated to fertility planning strategies. Their patterns of method and programme usage are not known. It seems unlikely that they can be encouraged to other patterns of use and discontinuation until more is known about their existing practices. A re-examination of current research categories will probably lead, as in the case of so-called 'reasons for discontiuation', to the realization that current tabulations and correlations are interpreted according to untested and untestable inferences. Exploration is needed to identify the relevant socio-cultural categories in local areas.

CHAPTER III: WHAT HAPPENS AFTER TERMINATION?

Previous chapters have traced the main influences on our understanding of the problem of discontinuation, noting the way in which research traditions have developed. The analysis has identified three activities which provide a rudimentary framework within which to examine information on 'drop-out' behaviour:-

(a) identifying simple record-keeping procedures for patterns of contraceptive use over time;

(b) reconsidering intervening variables with reference to the social and cultural specificity of the communities in which programmes operate; and

(c) reordering programme services and record-keeping procedures to fit the local patterns of contraceptive use identified by (a) and (b).

The present chapter considers possible methods of monitoring contraceptive use patterns, and the implications of a broader view of discontinuation for programme organization and evaluation. Attention is directed first to what is known of method changes, including a review of the various research techniques which have been used to derive this information. This suggests that patterns of use involving several methods are prevalent and can have considerable contraceptive effect, but that a more suitable data base is needed than that provided by use-effectiveness and acceptability studies.

The purpose of identifying patterns of continuation and discontinuation is to see whether they indicate segments of the ever-practising population most in need of family planning services. A number of problems related to method changes - users changing from one contraceptive source to another, method restarts, abortion, short-term discontinuation, and loss to follow-up - may be easier to understand and deal with when information on contraceptive use patterns becomes available. Obviously patterns of discontinuation, together with these related topics, are influenced positively or negatively by many aspects of family planning programmes. A review of the role of clinic factors in discontinuation shows that negative influences are not at present well understood; a different concept of discontinuation is needed to tackle these issues, and may lead to alterations in the way programmes are currently evaluated.

1 *Method Changes*

Method change data are irregularly reported and even then with a tendency to note only percentages of users adopting other contraceptives. Table V lists ten studies in eight countries, covering users who are either continuing a first method or practising a second at the time of study. A defect in this information is that the period or portion of the sample referred to is not always clear. In no case is the final drop-out category fully analysed to determine the extent of discontinuers still at risk. User success or failure with the second method is not regularly reported, nor whether the second method was the only alternative tried. The overall pattern suggests that more discontinuers will try a second method than not, but more will drop out than make a second attempt with the same method.

A detailed examination of one study can be used to show how the meaning of percentages is open to interpretation. The question is whether information reported in this form is sufficiently complete and clear to direct subsequent programme activities.

Freedman et. al. (90) in reporting a sample of

6,726 women in Taichung who accepted the IUD in the period July 1962 to December 1965 cite the following figures:

47.4 retained their original IUD;

7.9 had reinsertions;

17.7 adopted other methods or sterilization;

4.0 had abortions.

Thus, 77% of the couples were still practising contraception or had used abortion to prevent further births and 55% were still using an IUD.

These percentages can be interpreted in another way, to show that the major factor in the Taiwanese situation might be multiple use patterns rather than prevalence of the IUD. The 23 percent remaining unprotected consists of 11.2 percent pregnant and 11.8 percent not pregnant. Whether or not these women became or desired to become pregnant when the study was conducted, they are possible further users of contraception. It would be interesting to know what methods they subsequently adopted, and how soon after giving birth.

A later study (214) of 5,832 Taichung women, who accepted IUDs from July 1962 to May 1965 analyses their contraceptive use over a 6 to 9 year period. There is a further drop out, even allowing for reinsertions, of 21% of users continuing beyond a four year period. These women are proven continuers, though a number of them will have reached the end of their fertile period. This long-term study also shows an increase in the use of alternative methods: about 14% choose the pill or traditional methods, and about 19% are sterilized.

A crude comparison of first-method and several-method users may be gained by adding totals for known method changes (33%), abortions (4%) and the currently unprotected (23%). The resulting figure of 60% no doubt includes some later IUD returners, some menopausal women, and some who do not desire or need protection; on the other hand, it probably underestimates the number of abortions. Nonetheless it provides a useful contrast to the figures for IUD continuation (55% or 34% respectively) derived from the two studies. In areas which have not adopted Taiwan's emphasis on the IUD, the significance of post-termination events may be even greater.

Freedman, Jain and Sun (92) use regression techniques on the Taiwan data for further analysis of post-termination behaviour. They attempt to separate the socio-demographic correlates of: (i) continuing use with the IUD or some other method; (ii) continuation with a different method following IUD termination; and (iii) abortions subsequent to IUD use. The three categories are presented as a general gradation from use to discontinuation and pregnancy. The authors identify less educated and rural women who want to limit births, but who are without prior contraceptive experience as needing programme attention; there is a definite tendency for their pregnancies to be terminated in abortions. The authors suggest that these women are unaware of alternatives and should be followed up. Although the paper scarcely considers 'spacers', it also concludes that 'little can be gained by investing extra efforts among those women who accepted the IUD for spacing their births'.

This paper has the advantage of following a strategy of identifying continuing users, method changers, and discontinuers in an attempt to identify points of programme intervention. However, the data are organized in the format criticized above: a combination of standard socio-demographic variables according to common-sense inferences which, while plausible, are not really tested in the analysis. The quality and utility of their results are thus an interesting test of whether detailed information in a different form is really needed.

The study is restricted by three important premises. First, it effectively confines itself to 'limiters', setting aside those users who are not persistent family planners. (One may wonder whether all Taiwanese who were asked if they used contraception to limit or to space their children actually practise family planning in an either/or fashion).

This restriction could be made good by comparing how limiting strategies are practised within the three categories; however this requires more than correlating isolated socio-demographic characteristics with family planning behaviour. Hence a second limitation is that the significance of users' attributes identified in the study cannot be understood because of the way they are abstracted from the social processes to which they refer.

For example, IUD continuers are identified by the following attributes: satisfaction with the IUD, some prior contraceptive experience, and higher education. Method changers have the same characteristics, except that they are dissatisfied with the IUD. Additionally, they are urban, less than 35 years old, have some abortion experience, terminate in expulsion, and have reached their desired number of children (particularly of sons).

'Dissatisfaction with the IUD' is the only clear dividing factor between continuers and changers. The additional variables associated with the latter do not help us to understand this factor. There is not even the usual predominance of removals to suggest dissatisfaction. Those who continue are satisfied, those who do not are not satisfied: indeed, the authors note that 'there could be some circularity in this relationship'. Any informative difference between single and multiple method patterns collapses with this tautology.

The third limitation follows from the previous two. Since the study excludes spacing strategies, and does not effectively isolate method changes, the only group for which recommendations can be made are those non-continuers likely to abort. The study thus loses the advantages of comparing, for example, alternative strategies already being practised by similar women. What we want to know is why some limiters abort while others do not. The data show that the abortion group is like the method changers, except that they are younger, already have more children than they want, and are less educated. More urban residents have abortions, but rural terminators are more likely to have abortions. The authors are required to make an additional inference about user 'awareness' of alternatives, in order to combine these variables; but we still know very little about users' practice - in particular whether 'lack of awareness' is due to ignorance of family planning services, or to some other aspects of daily life. There remain rural and urban limiters with and without information who do and do not abort. The authors note that:

> "a proper study of whether or not abortion was used should consider whether or not contraception was used effectively during the preceding pregnancy interval. Unfortunately we do not have such sequential data about contraception and abortion in this sample."

Multiple variable techniques lend themselves to sorting out specific groups; some conventional variables such as age, parity and place of residence can probably be made informative if prior qualitative studies are used to increase the sophistication of inferences and variables (140). More thought should be given for example to questions such as whether 'urban/rural' is as relevant as locally recognized geographical, ethnic, or economic divisions; parity may be less relevant than gender preferences. The value of combinatory techniques depends entirely on the informativeness of the chosen variables and the extent to which they reflect factors operating at the local level.

Retrospective surveys, and user/non-user comparisons are other methods which might be considered appropriate for determining patterns of contraceptive use and discontinuation and related information. Westoff and Ryder (365) give an admirable critique of retrospective surveys as exemplified by the United States National Fertility Studies of 1965 and 1970. They trace broad trends in the extent of unwanted fertility, but their other basic finding is, as one might expect, that 'unwanted pregnancy' is a rather elastic concept, i.e. it stretches to fit changes in the perceived values of pregnancies. They complain that 'key questions on wanted and unwanted births yielded non-committal responses'. Their conviction that the extent of unwanted fertility is under-estimated is really a statement that 'elastic' concepts cannot be accurately measured. Two considerations enter here. First, survey responses made at any particular time are not necessarily valid for an entire fertile period whether for the individual or for a generation. Second, it is unrealistic to assume that respondents have firmly defined ideas or aspirations regarding their fertility. Patterns of adjustment are the matters of interest, and Westoff and Ryder state their preference for longitudinal information.

Inquiry into prior contraceptive practice may, like the question of unwanted pregnancies, be an inquiry into past sex life, marital stability and happiness, and the like. An individual's ability to recall sequences of use and discontinuation, the nature of present contraceptive practice, and change in the nature and availability of services all affect his response to questioning. Retrospective inquiries require an elaborate methodology and would need to be conducted regularly in order to provide data on use sequences. The likelihood of repeating a survey with the same sample is in many areas of the world very small.

Once data on use patterns becomes available, retrospective interviews may increase understanding of influences behind the patterns and of the extent to which identifiable sequences denote similar user experiences. The user's own perceptions of her past contraceptive practice may be very informative about the kind of service she now needs.

Another research strategy which appears in the study of differential contraceptive use is comparison of users and non-users. It is questionable whether patterns of use can be differentiated so simply, given the prevalence of discontinuation and of returns to contraception. 'User' and 'non-user' categories are too variegated to make it clear what is being compared. The same argument may be made for the comparison of 'user' and 'drop-out' categories: they are likely to contain the same people.

We can now turn to reports which contain information on method changes. Differences in the number and type of available methods are likely to have very different consequences for programmes, and this throws further doubt upon the significance of single method studies of acceptance and continuation. Where information is available, changes are usually recorded among three categories: oral, IUD and "other" methods. Table V suggests that changers represent between 14 and 65% of terminators, and terminators up to 75% of initial pill users in two years. Medical-related reasons for discontinuation seem to predominate among both changers and drop-outs. Information on abortion and sterilization is rare, and in many programmes only three or fewer method categories are currently utilized (202).

Ebanks (74) analyzed method changes up to the fourth attempt for two programmes in Barbados. One was the local Family Planning Association, newly promoting oral contraceptives; the other was a special project supported by the Population Council, newly promoting the IUD. Prior to the introduction of orals and the IUD, Barbadian women made fairly extensive use of vaginal methods: about 21% had prior contraceptive experience, mostly with these methods. Users tended to join the programme at first simply for cheaper supplies. Thus the first programme methods adopted most by women were vaginal methods. The subsequent pattern is more complex:

> "... predicting the second method used by a woman increases when her first method is known. The probability of accepting a vaginal method is the highest in all cases except where the first method was a vaginal, in which case it is the pill that is most frequently chosen in the BFPA sample and the IUD in the PCRP... In the BFPA sample, if the second method is a vaginal, the condom or an IUD, there is a high probability that the third method will be the pill. If the second method is the diaphragm or the pill, then the third method is likely to be a vaginal. In the PCRP sample of women the most likely third method of contraception is the IUD except in the case where the IUD was the second method, in which case it is either a vaginal or the pill. In changing from method 3 to method 4 ... the number of women involved ... is ... small ..."

The reason given most frequently for changes from first to second methods in both samples is desire for a more satisfactory method; second changes show a marked increase in reports of medical complaints, implying increased use of the pill and IUD; for the third and fourth method changes medical complaints predominate. Pregnancies over the same period decline. The overall change favours the clinically more effective methods.

Ebanks identifies several different patterns of use. Some women adopt a particular method, often their first, and use it consistently, whether it is the pill, a vaginal method, or an IUD. Harewood (102) confirms this pattern in Trinidad and Tobago for the pill, condoms and the IUD; similar patterns may occur in other areas. Harewood also notes a general trend toward more effective methods. A second group drops out after trying their first method, often in the first months of use: this is a very widespread pattern associated with orals and IUDs.

A further group, called 'changers' are the users referred to in the above quotation. Later studies (308, 349) show that the general situation described by Ebanks in 1968 still exists. These findings allow some explanation of method changes. Younger Barbadian women enter into a number of 'visiting unions' with a strong motive for avoiding pregnancy which varies according to change or absence of partners. The factor of 'visiting unions' implicitly explains continuing use of vaginal methods, method changes to and from vaginal methods and the low level of male involvement in contraceptive decision-making.

Laing (183) also provides more data on method changes than is usual. Of 1,865 completed interviews in the Philippines National Acceptor Survey, 391 (21%) record method changes in the first year. Drop-outs account for 14% of IUD acceptors, 34% of pill acceptors, and almost 50% of other methods. Laing does not describe method-by-method changes, but indicates trends which contrast with those noted by Ebanks. First segment pill users are more likely to change to rhythm or withdrawal, than to the IUD. More than half of IUD terminators select the pill, and one-fourth adopt rhythm and withdrawal. Women changing from rhythm are likely to adopt the pill. Laing concludes that 'the quality of the later method tended to be considerably poorer than the quality of the first method'.

Reasons for terminating a first method are mostly for 'side-effects' which Laing notes cannot be separately determined. 'Accidental pregnancy' is the second most frequent reason, though predominant for rhythm. Medical factors (33.4%) are the most important single reason for terminating the most recent method but pregnancy and planned pregnancy together make up 41.6% of the total. Continuation is higher among progressively older women of higher parity; husbands' opinions and prior exposure to family planning are cited as deciding factors.

These two examples show that data which follow method shifts change by change, rather than by first and last methods used, give a clearer idea of audience segmentation over time, indicating patterns of return to the oral or IUD after various changes and perhaps pregnancies. Do younger women who have had medical and related complaints with these methods return to them as they increasingly approach older age and higher parity? Or will they turn to abortion, sterilization or large families?

The patterns described in these studies suggest that dropping-out is likely to follow method changes in which the user remains dissatisfied, thus including not only women disenchanted with modern methods in the first months of their experience, but women who are willing to make more than one attempt, and with more than one method.

Method change data suggest that explanation of contraceptive use in terms of the motivated/unmotivated dichotomy, like that of limiters/spacers, over-simplifies the longitudinal experience of contraceptive use. These distinctions are really just convenient ways of circumscribing the number of variables to be studied, but they tend to become objects of study themselves, and thus get in the way of understanding specific, local situations. The opposite findings in the two studies with regard to spouses' participation, trends towards more or less effective methods, and the different methods that come to be used consistently are a reminder of cultural and programme variation.

There can be little doubt of the desirability of increasing changes to more effective methods, but more must be known about the nature of method changes generally. As younger groups increase in numbers due to the age distribution of most Third World populations, the patterns of use and discontinuation of multiple methods may influence an increasingly important amount of fertility, according to the pace at which initially dissatisfied users settle-down to particular patterns of contraceptive use with particular methods. It would be interesting to know what proportion of clinic case loads is represented by users of, say, more than two methods, and what intervals separate each adoption of a contraceptive. As will be shown in Chapter IV, a systematic approach is needed to monitor this information.

2 *Some Related Issues in a Multi-Method Context*

Little information is available for what might be called sub-topics of the multi-method issue: use of different contraceptive services; reinsertion and method restarts; abortion; short-term discontinuation; and loss to follow-up. The implications of each of these topics will be considered separately.

There have been several recent requests (49, 93, 267) for further attention to the 'substitution effect' which in this case refers to users who 'drop-out' of a family planning programme, but go on practising with the same or other methods obtained from different sources. Substitution of sources presents several problems. There is evidence (64, 74, 181) that some users discontinue because they consult several clinic organizations, receiving varying advice and methods. It may in such circumstances become difficult for a consistent pattern to develop. Cobliner et. al. (64) note that these women tend to become abortion repeaters.

Special distribution projects, co-ordinated with or by family planning programmes, and often using regular retail outlets are a recent attempt to bridge the gap between conventional clinic programmes and commercial marketing (9, 69, 79, 114, 256). They have received added emphasis from recent decisions favouring oral pill distribution without medical examinations and prescription[6]. Projects of this kind can reach much more extensive rural areas than is possible at present with clinics alone, and the use of indigenous networks also makes contraception culturally more acceptable. Moreover, because some of these projects work on an inter-personal level, method use, discontinuation and change can be monitored for individuals and groups (79). Where clinics, community based distribution and commercial sources are all under one head, it may be possible to assess the extent of method source substitution.

The picture of reinsertions (1, 51, 78, 89, 90, 92, 107, 153, 169, 213, 236, 302) and oral contraceptive restarts (50, 125, 132, 349, 361, 380) seems reasonably clear. Detailed data on reinsertion are available

---

6 International Planned Parenthood Federation, Central Medical Committee on the Distribution of Oral Contraceptives. Statement issued April, 1973

mostly on Taiwan, and indicate that most IUD users who reinsert have experienced expulsions; for example, in the Taichung Medical Follow-up (89), 65% of expulsions led to reinsertion, compared to only 12% of terminations for all other reasons. These studies indicate that discontinuation of reinsertions follows the same overall pattern as first insertions. Reinsertion thus makes a moderate but significant contribution to IUD continuation, particularly for those women who have had their first IUD for longer periods.

Since most oral contraceptive discontinuers stop for medical or personal reasons related to side-effects, restarts are analogous to reinsertions following voluntary removal of IUDs. Oral restarts have not been the primary subject of studies as have reinsertions; nor have restarts following experimentation with other methods, or delayed restarts. Such studies may only become feasible as attention turns to sequential use patterns.

Data on abortion are known to be inaccurate and under-reported. Abortion would seem fundamentally related to 'limiting' patterns determined by age and parity, as suggested by the 1966 Taiwan IUD follow-up (92), and may be an indicator of dissatisfaction with contraceptive methods.

But do drop-outs regularly resort to abortion, and if so, what kind of use patterns do they represent? Abortion rarely figures in family planning as a programme method, but two hypotheses often appear: that increased contraception reduces abortion by reducing pregnancies, or that it increases the number of abortions because of heightened commitment to limitation. Estimates of the percentage of discontinuers subsequently using abortion are available for only a few countries, notably Korea (137, 138, 358, 275, 164, 90, 273), but suggest that abortion is indeed an important component of contraceptive practice.

A general picture emerges from Tietze and Mursteins' review (348). Abortion is an inevitable component of the multi-method situation. Increases in use of contraception and abortion appear to go together, so that both hypotheses apply. As more and more women adopt contraception, and have mixed experiences with it, they make up more and more of the population likely to experience an unwanted pregnancy. There may or may not be a link between the two trends and further research is indicated.

It seems likely that current interpretations of abortion figures contain artifacts due to classification. For example, those who resort to abortion tend to be classified as 'contraceptive failures', rather than as users who for some reason prefer abortion. Studies of abortion repeaters (64, 148, 149, 260, 316) suggest that the psychological situation of women who become pregnant despite the availability of contraceptives they know how to use is much more subtle than the simple category 'contraceptive failure' allows. The segments of the using or not-using population under consideration are however difficult to specify using current methods.

It may be expected that a considerable number of those who abort are high parity women who are 'limiters', or those in the youngest age groups not wanting any children at present. What are their patterns of previous contraceptive use and at what points in their contraceptive histories, particularly in the older groups, do breaks-in-use appear? Do abortions follow closely on contraceptive discontinuance? Women who use abortion could help us to understand the 'limiting' ideology of family planning. Of equal interest are those women who use abortion for spacing, or without any apparent family planning strategy.

More immediate gains in knowledge seem possible for two other topics pertaining to breaks in use, viz. short-term discontinuation and loss to follow-up. Relatively simple alterations in clinic routine may affect the extent of loss in these categories.

A number of studies report pill 'acceptors' who never begin use (80, 130, 132, 138, 366, 381); drop-out in the first three cycles is also a familiar pattern of oral discontinuation (147, 275, 306). The problem is related to the question of irregular usage of oral contraceptives and coitus-related methods. A recent review noted that the 'current level of knowledge about contraceptive compliance and factors in compliance is very limited', and that both prediction of noncompliance and developments in contraceptive technology await better data (119).

Sear and Turner (293) have written the only published paper on short term discontinuation. Among 405 oral contraceptive acceptors in a New Orleans, Louisiana family planning clinic, 5.2% did not take the pills, largely because of menstrual irregularities which led to an inability to determine when to begin use. An additional 6.1% stopped during or immediately after the first cycle, principally due to break-through bleeding. The authors note that these apparently small groups could account for as much as two-fifths of first year discontinuation. As use sequences are not at issue for these groups, they comprise an immediately distinguishable pattern of discontinuation.

The potential importance of those lost to follow-up would seem to be a closed topic: after all, if they are 'lost' there is little that can be said about them. The standard procedure (357) is simply to apportion them to relevant groups according to demographic characteristics, or by randomization. This is really a recipe for forgetting that they exist.

Studies which list in some detail why a sample was incompletely covered (7, 152, 183, 216, 236, 317, 350) conform to a pattern; the overwhelming cause is related to user location (no address in records; wrong address; moved); the remaining reasons, usually refusal or temporary absence, make up something less than 10% of the loss. Many studies exclude follow-up of geographically distant users for reasons of time or cost. Data processing often wastes information by combining categories in order to facilitate coding. Finally, special causes often preclude data collection altogether - for example, Laing notes armed conflict in Muslim areas of the Philippines (183), and similar cases could be noted for other countries.

Those lost to follow up are important because they are particularly likely to be at risk of pregnancy: giving a wrong or inadequate address is a well-known sign of ambivalence about family planning; distance from source of supply may discourage use. Cultural and psychological factors are the most likely to be eliminated in data processing, or analysis. For example, cultural, linguistic and social factors relevant to the conduct of interviews are given little attention in the literature.

Most of these factors are to some extent unavoidable, although their influence should be noted. Studies frequently report author's opinions that bias due to LFU is not significant; sometimes this refers to statistical checks, and sometimes to the author's impression of the conduct of research. Rarely is the reader enabled to assess these statements, particularly regarding the nature of data collection. Social structural and cultural information on the communities studied is usually not recorded. Reports seldom indicate the extent of the main investigator's familiarity with the languages and peoples he or his staff are studying, though this may affect his capacity to find informants classified as 'lost'.

For example, is 'failure to give correct address' a problem because in conditions such as rapidly expanding West African towns or Latin American barrios, the notion of a personal 'address' is not particularly meaningful? Traditional village organization may specify residence through a variety of occupational, kinship or ritual identifications. It is sometimes suggested that if 'address' is inappropriate, the user should be asked to name someone through whom she could be contacted; in field studies it is advisable to note landmarks, directions etc. (272).

One way of lessening loss to follow-up may be to make better use of certain information resources. Heads of lineages or families, midwives, priests, shopkeepers, and so forth, are likely to know the households in their area, or know how to locate or find out about them. To identify a contact for follow-up it may be appropriate to ask such questions as: 'What is your husband's lineage?'; 'Who is your elder?'; 'From whom do you buy flour?'; 'Who delivered your last child?'

Attention to indigenous social networks may also be informative. If there is considerable movement and migration within and between communities, simple transfer arrangements between clinics (for example, identity cards, transferable coupons, special service cards) may be worth consideration. These geographical movements may be related to other factors, such as unstable conjugal unions. Changes of partners may account for inaccuracies in names or husbands' names in clinic records. Finally, audience segmentation according to patterns of use and discontinuation may reveal a pattern of loss to follow-up, because smaller studies carried out on particular segments are likely to allow more intensive coverage than in large randomized surveys.

In short, better attention to and reduction of losses to follow-up seems likely to result from better research design, higher standards of reporting and better knowledge of the community before research begins.

3 *What Happens in the Clinic?*

Before turning to the problems of understanding patterns of contraceptive use and disuse in specific contexts, writings on programme procedures which may be a negative influence on continuation must be reviewed. No one would argue that clinic conditions are without influence on users, nor that even their most ordinary activities are identical in value from one society to the next. Yet the influence of clinic-related factors on continuation has received much less attention than method and socio-demographic factors. We do not know whether manipulation of clinic variables would decrease user dissatisfaction among discontinuers who experience bleeding, pain and other 'side-effects' or who are not settling down to a particular method.

The problem described for use-effectiveness research arises again in clinic studies (33, 36, 44, 65, 68, 94, 97, 141, 142, 144, 205, 208, 219, 220, 258, 261, 268, 290, 292, 294, 301, 309, 317, 319, 320, 360, 362). The net-rate life table approach is inapplicable since the forces behind discontinuation are not simply additive but multiple, and of different kinds. No convincing framework for clinic studies has emerged and almost every one of these articles defines the important issues and parameters differently.

These studies have inherited much of the socio-demographic and medical methodology of use-effectiveness studies. Some papers on programme or clinic discontinuation refer only to methods and stereo-typed reasons (141, 258, 268, 309, 317, 370). Almost all studies of clinic influence, however, find that the reasons most often given for dropping out are method-related. The socio-demographic categories for clinic discontinuation conform to the same high parity and older age classifications as for method discontinuation

(35, 208, 219, 319). This is useful baseline data, but no straightforward plan of action can be expected from it. Attempts to compile clinic discontinuation rates, perhaps in order to contrast with method discontinuation rates, have not met with success (36, 68).

Clinic discontinuation studies have not reconsidered the prevailing framework for studying contraceptive use. The argument seems to be that although clinic-related factors are more than or at least as important as method complaints, a separate research strategy is not required to study them. Some of the writings most concerned with clinic effects (35, 68, 142, 261) are those which distinguish method from clinic drop-outs by listing method-related and clinic-related 'reasons' in separate tables. An ambiguous set of 'reasons' for method discontinuation has been supplemented by additional clinic variables; the resulting combination is no easier to interpret. It is more than likely that most users could be classified into both sets.

There would however seem to be three cases for which a separation of predominantly method or clinic-related factors in discontinuation might be argued. One is the woman who comes into the clinic or is informed of family planning in some systematic way, but does not take up a method. She is of interest as a non-user and not as a drop-out. Although this aspect has received some attention (293, 304) it is not clear, except when women state their disapproval of family planning, what separates the never-user from the very short term user. If either has any previous contraceptive experience, non-use may be due to a factor such as the clinic's image in the community.

A second group of 'clinic drop-outs' are those women who subsequently obtain contraceptive supplies and services from another source. As indicated above, they are of interest as a data problem rather than a discontinuation problem: conventional ways are needed of identifying such women in order to assess the extent to which they make perhaps unnecessary demands on services. At present only percentages of acceptors are reported in this category - 12 per cent (35); 4 per cent (142); 11 per cent (214); 20 per cent (262).

In the third category are women who give clinic faults as a primary factor in discontinuation, for which estimates range from 17 to 47 per cent of new acceptors (35, 141, 144, 262). Medical complaints are also numerous, but the extent of overlap with service-related complaints is not explored. It is additionally very difficult to assess the significance of these studies, since the samples involved are frequently small: Bracken and Kasl (35) refer to a drop-out sample of 299 women; Reynolds (262) to 40 women eligible for contraception out of a sample of 60; and Mundigo (219) to 85 drop-outs.

Some studies take up the possibility that clinic factors rather than socio-demographic or method variables determine the outcome of a user's continuing effort at pregnancy prevention in the first months of contraception (142, 219, 220, 319). Variations between clinics in the proportion of drop-outs in related areas suggests that services are the major factor. Clinic deficiences include: excessive waiting times; shortage of doctors; poor organization of patient flow through the clinic; excessive paper work; lack of interest among doctors; unsympathetic staff attitudes, particularly regarding linguistic, cultural or economic differences; lack of privacy; inadequate or over-elaborate contraceptive information; and supply shortages. However, the studies show that complaints about these factors cannot be correlated with discontinuation. Improvements in information services have no impact on continuation rates. Keller (142) concludes that 'factors unmeasured in the present study probably influence desertion (sic) levels by clinic in conjunction with some or all of the measured ones'.

The measures typically used in clinic discontinuation research apply to clinic effects on users without reference to marital, familial, sexual or other indigenous patterns of which contraception may be a mere adjunct. Reports that institutional and convenience factors are not a reason for discontinuation (205), that user complaints do not necessarily lead to discontinuation (95, 142), or that variables such as patient/staff ratios, number of patients per medical hour, etc., do not correlate with drop-outs (142, 320) probably reflect the inadequacy of the measures used. Measuring operational variables is not the same as measuring users' clinic experience.

The quality and utility of these findings are so similar to those of use-effectiveness studies that many of the same criticisms apply. Social and cultural backgrounds are not explored. The character of interviews and interviewers is not reported. Research is concentrated on first method discontinuation, scarcely touching upon post-termination events. Crucial factors in the individual's perception of family planning, such as the way he or she learns to describe bodily experiences or to handle encounters with public health or other institutions, are also ignored. Diverse, isolated statements are interpreted as comparable 'reasons' for discontinuation despite the different values attached by users to experiences in the clinic, between husband and wife, within a woman's reference group, and so forth. Statements taken out of context in order to fit a largely predetermined set of inferences are not of much practical use in accounting for programme events.

These studies however, document some of the worst fears about inefficient or insensitive clinic procedures. Evaluations of these procedures - patient flow through the clinic, comparative efficiency of information techniques, etc. - are certainly worth doing for administrative purposes. However, any attempt to measure 'clinic discontinuation' as a separate but in some sense analogous phenomenon to 'method discontinuation' is surely a red herring. The point of clinic studies must be to discern the principal cultural, social and psychological factors inherent in clinical procedures which influence contraceptive use patterns.

It is likely to be very difficult to identify long-term discontinuers on the basis of unfavourable clinic experiences. The advantages of identifying certain clinic procedures as sources of difficulty are tied to specific instances. Even when continuing clinic shortcomings can be identified, they do not necessarily have a direct and consistent influence upon contraceptive continuation.

This raises an important question for family planning evaluation, particularly in relation to more recent developments, such as community based distribution projects, which have thus far been evaluated in a use-effectiveness framework (9, 69). While writers agree that programmes should be organized to fit local conditions and cultural preferences (9, 69, 79, 114, 256) with increasing use of non-or para-medical personnel (26, 234, 266, 267, 269, 270, 378, 386), little has been published about the type of evaluation required to judge programmes based on these different premises. How can evaluation best reflect the indigenous values and preferences which shape user experiences?

Scrimshaw's study of women's reactions to a family planning clinic in Guayaquil, Ecuador provides a useful example (290). Her survey of some three thousand women was preceded by anthropological fieldwork, which identified customary modes of thought and action related to concepts of female modesty and shame, health and illness, and to womanhood and the place of women in society. On this basis Scrimshaw makes a number of direct recommendations on the treatment of women in clinics: interviews, pelvic examinations, and areas for dressing and undressing should be private; medical examinations should require minimum physical exposure; the examinations should be as simple and uncluttered by extraneous questions as possible; frequency of examinations and supply visits should be kept to a minimum; and female personnel should be employed wherever possible.

The argument that social codes of behaviour, such as those referring to modesty, can be identified and acted upon in specific programme activities has important implications. Community-based contraceptive distribution, and projects involving traditional midwives already tacitly recognize local patterns of behaviour. If indigenous morality can be used to guide programmes, it may also be the best basis for evaluation. This is a major departure from current programme evaluation in several senses.

First, it means that organizing principles are shared between the community and the programme. This applies as well to the organization of research. Surveys, already informed by local rules of behaviour, should be used to measure the extent to which programme activities are seen as coherent and positive by the local population.

Secondly, it suggests that family planning programmes need not be judged simply by numbers of new acceptors or by the length of first method use. We have already pointed out that several different patterns of contraceptive continuation and discontinuation are likely to exist in communities, and that it is unrealistic to evaluate programmes on the basis of one (rather idealised) pattern of long-term use. Patterns of continuation and discontinuation are obviously a product of both indigenous and programme influences, and both sources of contraceptive practise need to be taken into account. Modesty and embarrassment in the clinic are good examples: lessening the emotional stress of clinic situations may be a desirable and important programme objective in itself. Programme activities might well be judged on such a basis, provided it is recognized that the specific causes and consequences can be expected to vary in different cultures.

Third, understanding the values of a community has a direct bearing on the interaction between users and programme personnel. This interaction is not merely inter-personal: a wide range of cultural facts may be called upon by both users and staff to interpret each others' actions, whether they belong to the same community or not. These facts are likely to be more practical and informative than the advice that 'what really counts is having someone who is sympathetic to talk to' (44).

This quotation suggests that many difficulties encountered in clinics can be overcome by personal sensitivity, together with a good dose of common sense. It is important to point out how variable common sense and sensitivity can be. It seems self-evident that women would not want to be questionned on their sex lives or to have medical examinations in public.

Yet such things happen, as Scrimshaw points out, in societies with elaborate and emotionally powerful codes of modesty. Customary beliefs and behaviour about menstruation in many Muslim and Hindu areas may mean that women who experience irregular bleeding patterns with the pill or IUD cannot cook, move about, or sleep with their husbands. How should staff handle women whose complaints of bleeding are, by implication, requests to be removed from a state of ritual impurity? How much should women be told about the usual side-effects of the pill and IUD?

In summary, it is fair to say that the question of organizational influences on patterns of contraceptive use is perhaps the most wide-open and unresolved of the whole topic of discontinuation. Attempts to find consistent links between programme organization drop-outs have been frustrated by a multitude of possible factors and hampered by a not very helpful distinction between method and clinic-related reasons for discontinuation. Little attention has been given to post-termination behaviour or to devising specific clinic procedures to cope with method-related problems such as side-effects. This situation will continue while narrow evaluative criteria of continuation and organizational efficiency are adhered to. Much of the interaction of users with programme staff and organization cannot be fairly judged in terms of continuation. As programmes become more directed to the needs and lives of users and adapted to the characteristics of the communities they serve, different methods of evaluating them from this point of view must be found.

CHAPTER IV: A METHOD FOR RECORDING TYPES OF DISCONTINUATION

The preceding chapters have shown that discontinuation has rarely been studied for its own distinctive features as a regular and foreseeable aspect of family planning. The category 'drop-out' covers a diverse group of people many of whom are still practising contraception, but the composition of which is largely unknown. This chapter addresses the explanatory aspect of the problem, that is, the issue of selecting the variables appropriate to finding out who drops out and why.

In the absence of data on patterns of use and discontinuation, a typology of eight patterns is hypothesized, according to several assumptions. It seems likely that only a minority of women adopt from the beginning of their reproductive period the basic ideology of long-term contraceptive planning promoted by family planning organizations. Patterns of use may be viewed as a process through which certain women learn this ideology or its equivalent, not so much by being taught, as by physical, emotional and mental experience. Women who see themselves as limiters may or may not achieve this in practice, but it seems unlikely that extended and successful contraception over several years will occur without the emergence of some definite pattern of use.

Nonetheless, we need a way of describing women who practise contraception, though not for the purpose of family limiting purposes. In some cases 'spacing' may be an adequate concept for this group, but not, for example, for most young unmarried women in the English speaking world. It is likely that many languages have no equivalent concept. To start with, it seems simple enough just to say that most women practise birth control because at a given moment they do not want to get pregnant. These can be called 'short-term users', and those who express and attempt strategies such as limiting and spacing, 'long-term users'. The final premise is that there is a natural tendency for short-term users, as they gain in experience and grow older, to see themselves as long term users. Continuous use, then, embraces whatever methods and combinations of methods over time facilitate development of this capability.

The objective of a typology of contraceptive practice is not crisp categorization, but a general sorting of users into groups of greater or lesser priority. It should also suggest programme efforts needed for each category. It is of the utmost importance to let a classification such as the following guide exploration of possible types. Rather than imposed as a set of preconceived ideas, a typology may be successively modified until it aptly describes the pattern of events of interest. It is a means to new and culturally specific definitions of discontinuation. Having set out some rough types, we can then turn to how a typology is used as a discovery procedure to develop appropriate information about priority groups.

A *Short-term users*. These are men or women who attach varying priority to contraceptive practice. Generally, other aspects of their lives appear to be more compelling than regulation of fertility. Thus a woman may take up a contraceptive method because she does not want at present to get pregnant, but this may be effectively less important to her than cultural and psychological factors associated with the role of women in society. No spacing strategy need be involved, for in many cultures this concept is unknown; nor is it likely to be applicable in many societies during the early and most fecund period of marriage. Three subdivisions may be suggested

(i) *method changers:* who change to or from the IUD and oral, which remain the principal methods in many programmes. Information is required on the incidence of physical complaints and on readoption of methods. Method changes may suggest that better support and information about method effects is needed by the user; efforts to maintain continuation on an alternate method may be necessary. The length of time a user tries a method before stopping may be especially significant. There is an obvious interest in whether the method change patterns becomes a limiting pattern (number (v) below). The question also arises as to whether the cafeteria approach encourages 'frivolous' method changes - i.e. before a method has really been given its due.

(ii) *sporadic users:* who use contraception irregularly for personal and social reasons. Local conditions may account for this pattern, such as marital instability, or a prevalence of visiting unions.

(iii) *immediate discontinuers:* who never use the method they have 'accepted', or do so for a very short time. This interval may be set at whatever point seems significant in the year following initial use. It seems likely that physical-related problems with the IUD and pill, aesthetic problems with traditional methods, and information failures on the part of programmes are all at issue here.

B *Long-term users.* These are men or women with well-formed childbearing strategies which accord with programme goals of extended use, who may realistically be called 'family planners'. Both 'limiting' and 'spacing' strategies, and a variety of methods or abortion may be used. An important question is at what point in their contraceptive histories they adopt this pattern. Do they become 'limiters' or 'spacers'? The following sub-divisions presume this distinction, but may be replaced by local alternatives.

(iv) who continue with their first method throughout their contraceptive life span. This group also might contain those who, having consistently used one method, are then sterilised.

(v) who try several methods, perhaps including abortion, but settle down to a particular method. Incidence of physical-related complaints, the sequence of different methods and gaps, and the availability of options and services are all likely to be important for this group.

(vi) who do not or who have not yet consistently limited, or who allow lengthy unprotected periods to occur when they are aware of some contraceptive methods. These women may have a history of abortion. Psychological and cultural factors are likely to be important, since the means-ends strategy of patterns (iv) and (v) no longer applies. This group may be significantly large.

Spacers:

(vii) who continue with their first method, and return to it after a pregnancy.

(viii) who do not settle down to a consistent pattern of method use. The interest of separating these spacer categories is to find out whether the expressed intention to space has anything to do with consistent practice; whether for example, women in both categories will eventually become limiters, and whether there is any difference in the number of births before a limiting strategy is adopted. The expectation, of course, is that continuous use and a return to contraception shortly after giving birth are significant in their effects; this suggests that self-described spacers are an important audience.

A typology is an audience segmentation strategy, not an end in itself. It should be revisable, and it can be expected to change as more and more is known about discontinuers, or as the community changes. We should be suspicious of neatly itemized sets of discontinuation types, for there is no reason to expect that all users will conform to the most frequently occurring patterns. Nor is there any reason to insist that the patterns are altogether natural, that is, in some sense existing without the discovery procedure. Programmes need to develop models for their own purposes, and a typology of discontinuation serves mainly two purposes:

> (a) to divide up the overall target population, allowing a manageable number of sub-groups to be selected for further attention; and (b) to provide for identified priority groups a fairly strong indication of their problems and interests.

In developing this strategy, programmes need to draw as heavily as possible upon knowledge of daily life in local communities, for these cultural contexts set the conditions under which programmes operate.

Procedures for developing a typology may be divided into a review and a follow-up. It is assumed that the investigator is someone familiar with a particular programme who has some intuition of likely patterns of discontinuation. The review stage is intended to make the most of available information and clinic records, or of information that may be derived by making a few minimal changes in recording procedures. The follow-up involves further studies which may be indicated by the review.

1 *Review of Available Information*

The most basic information may be collected with little more effort than is currently expended on clinic record systems. Manuals on clinic records, (99, 229, 262, 272) usually contain questions on current and past methods used, and sometimes on the date of changes. Gaps in clinic and contraceptive use have in the past been standardised by identifying users who have not returned for a check-up within three months as 'drop-outs', and removing them from active files. While this definition can be used in the first instance, an important question as study proceeds is whether this is a realistic procedure. It may be preferable to begin with ongoing operations, and for specified periods emphasize the recording of method changes, dates of changes and delayed returns to the clinic.

The advantage of using records systems is that changes in user status are recorded as they occur; the disadvantage is that many important changes in status, for example substitutions or gaps in use, may not be detected in the records. In some cases, samples already drawn from clinic records can be followed up by re-interviews. Previous surveys may be particularly informative about possible obstacles to follow-up. An investigator, having familiarised himself with available record or survey data and the methods used to collect it, will probably have revised or confirmed his first hypothesis of the contraceptive use patterns he is looking for, and whether and how the existing record system can be used to identify them.

Most patterns of use and discontinuation probably cannot be discerned simply from records, without reference to the material conditions and cultural specificity of local peoples. The process of determining types is one of coming to associate certain specific user problems and rationalizations with certain sorts of use sequence. The two sources of information are used to correct each other: the recorded sequences of use are an empirical check on the number of cultural factors to be considered; while local data serves to make some sense out of sequences of contraception, gaps in use, pregnancies, and so forth. For example, sporadic and unsuccessful limiter groups may be differentiated by different social patterns (visiting versus stable unions), even though stops and starts with various methods may look very similar in the records.

A review of information on the contexts of contraceptive discontinuation is necessitated by the inadequacy of previously applied methods and data on 'reasons for discontinuation'. The investigator's personal experience and familiarity with local values and constraints is a prerequisite for intelligent investigation. He must be aware of sources of influence often neglected in previous studies, e.g., unreported changes in personnel recording the information, conditions relating to the privacy of the interview, 'scares' or rumours, and significant political or economic events independent of the programme. Appreciating the significance of what may appear to be extraneous detail requires a definite awareness of local points of view, not simply on isolated topics but for their coherence as part of indigenous language and custom.

Cultural background can also be provided by reference to existing research on local communities, particularly anthropological studies, although much more work is needed to make these materials available to programme personnel. It will probably be necessary to include in the review of qualitative factors several open-ended discussions with appropriate programme personnel, users, and locally important figures.

The review thus has two components, record-keeping and a qualitative assessment. We can speculate briefly on the information produced by the review, and the audience segments it may identify for further attention. Adequate description of certain patterns of contraceptive use, and especially of programme action needed for them, will require further information derived from follow-up studies.

The records in themselves are likely to give rise to broad patterns, which then require internal differentiation. Aggregates of short term discontinuers and of steadfast continuers are probably separable in the first instance from the broad band of users with variable patterns.

Perhaps users who try more than one method (or patterns in the sequence of methods used) may be separated out of this middle group. A potential 'spacer' group might also be selected on the basis of a year or so of continuous contraception which ultimately is broken off. It would be interesting to find out how many of these women actually practice spacing as such i.e. who describe their contraceptive practise using that concept.

The main business of sorting out divisions within these groups can only be carried out on the basis of what users and services are known or thought to be like. Small numbers of extended or open interviews may be conducted after initial sorting and in terms of available information on cultural distinctions. These first interviews can be used for a number of purposes, particularly trying out culturally informed questions.

Several means of reconnaissance may be advisable where there is uncertainty about how best to phrase inquiries, or where interviews are likely to yield only information thought acceptable to the interviewer. Particularly adept field workers or clinic staff, or regular clinic users are important resources. Available information and knowledge of important cultural factors should be supplemented by the investigator's day to day contact with a community. The issue is not only how to translate questions into the local idiom, but to identify the questions already being asked and answered in the community.

A number of variable patterns are identified in the typology: v (limiters who used several methods before resolving upon one); vi and viii (limiters and spacers without a consistent method of preference); iii (short term users adopting a variety of methods); and ii (other sporadic short-term users). The first of these is of interest largely for comparative purposes; the second groups may also be of comparative interest with reference to immediate discontinuers, since both are likely to contain significant amounts of side-effects and method-related complaints. The group identified as 'sporadic' has already been noted as one guided by dominant social patterns independent of family planning, such as marital patterns or visiting unions. These women are not likely priorities for follow-up, but they are examples of users for whom provision of a variety of methods may be an important service. Other local factors which may underlie sporadic use are ritual prescriptions of various kinds (possibly related to ethnic identity) and migrant labour.

The interest in changer and spacer groups is to find out and ensure that these people are indeed in transitional stages prior to sustained use. The consistent ways in which gaps in use occur and how they are or are not coped with may have a great deal to do with whether a user gradually becomes a successful or unsuccessful limiter.

Thus, a typology makes it possible to give different priorities to different groups. Attention should be directed to limiters who are not in fact preventing births (pattern vi) and to others which lead to significant gaps in use (i, iii, viii). Some patterns (ii), although representing important audience segments, are unlikely to respond to special programme efforts. Short term discontinuers (iii) require different attention than those who may be considered sequentially, that is, those users who consider themselves in the process of changing methods or patterns and learning which contraceptives they prefer (vi, viii). Pattern (v), since it reflects the variable groups which seem to involve the majority of users, may be a much more realistic basis for programme evaluation than the currently used pattern (iv), which is simply a presumptive ideal. A programme may need to choose its priorities for follow-up between several potentially important groups.

2 *Follow-up*

The review should decide what types of follow-up are needed, what groups it is directed to, and what resources are available. Since the present study is directed to improving the information upon which programmes act, changes in follow-up services will not be considered here. The review is likely to indicate two kinds of further study which are needed: (a) to identify and understand which local factors are the significant constraints on particular groups of users; and (b) to confirm the factuality of the identified patterns.

In the first case, in-depth qualitative studies may be directed to particular groups identified by the typology. The potential significance of indigenous concepts of modesty, and of women's attitudes towards their bodies and to changing social roles has already been noted, as well as the significance of varying conjugal relationships. Community pressures having to do with family and economic organization may be powerful forces in discontinuation.[7] Traditional medical practices, which belong to a wider conceptual order embracing religion, nature, diet, sex, marriage and other areas of belief and practice, depending on the society, may be an important factor in influencing users.[8]

The main consideration is that local information is a different kind of information from that collected in surveys and records. It is a translation of the patterns and priorities of particular cultures, and can only claim to represent them fairly if it follows the order they lay down. We cannot credibly claim an interest in improving the lives and conditions of peoples

---

7 Jongmans, D.G. Socio-cultural Aspects of Family Planning: An Anthropological Study at the Village Level. In: The Neglected Factor. D.G. Jongmans, H.J.M. Claessen (eds). Pp. 33-66. 1974

8 Jocano, F.L. Cultural Changes in Relation to a Sustained Country-wide Family Planning Programme. International Planned Parenthood Federation, South East Asia and Oceania Region. Monograph No.2. Pp. 24. 1972

if our understanding of them is ordered solely by the patterns and priorities of surveys we have designed.[9]

Confirmation and correction of the typology may subsequently be carried out using survey methods. The investigator must decide whether a systematic random sample can be drawn from existing records, or from ongoing records to which questions on contraceptive use sequences have been added. A sample will be necessary since information contained in clinic records on user case histories will in many cases be incomplete. He will also need to decide whether the full range of users in the records should be sampled or only certain groups. Questions derived from intensive studies may thus be tested more widely.

In sum, the question arises whether patterns of use and discontinuation over time do indeed exist, and whether they correlate consistently with patterns of user experience. An audience segmentation strategy is needed for its ability to exclude sizeable ranges of the overall target population, identifying a workable number for attention; and to provide for identified priority groups a fairly strong indication of their problem and interests.

The idea of audience segmentation is hardly new, but is usually viewed in relation to new users. With reference to continuation, the two important benefits of the approach are: that it can be used as the basis for a discovery procedure which utilizes available data of several kinds; and that it enables a variety of comparisons to be made

---

9 More extensive consideration of important features of cultural information is contained in the Draft Report on which this monograph is based. See: Kreager, P. Discontinuation of Family Planning Methods and Programmes: Consultants Report. IPPF. November 1976.

,roups and users. The procedure is more realistic parisons of broad and ethnocentric categories such ters' and 'spacers' or 'motivated' and 'unmotivated'. It is not based on the too apparent objective of turning everyone as quickly as possible into well-motivated limiters. It thus may provide a more realistic basis for programme evaluation by leading to a more credible standard for user performance.

Patterns of use may, of course, be heavily influenced by recent promotional programmes or clinical preference for certain methods. This does not make them of less interest or value. On the one hand they may suggest that programme difficulties are a consequence of past failures such as lack of ready options for those women who dislike the pill and IUD. On the other hand, it may provide a constructive answer to the differential impact of promotional programmes, especially the discouraging results of some attempts (46, 320). There is, additionally, the interesting question of whether the acceptor in a heavily promoted campaign is in fact a good continuer. This no longer needs to be judged merely by first method longevity. In short, the typology suggests a way in which the injunction 'follow the user' may actually be taken up.

CHAPTER V: CONCLUSION

The perspective adopted in this review considers the problem of 'drop-outs' a normal aspect of patterns of contraceptive use. Discontinuation cannot come as a surprise: the natural side-effects of the principal contraceptives, and the differences between users, services and the societies to which they belong, are given features of any organized family planning service. The main problem seems to be one of faulty definition, which not only exaggerates the problem, but inhibits any attempts to deal with it.

The category 'drop-out' is so variegated that it is of little analytic or practical value. On close examination it encompasses those who are and are not presently practising contraception, those who do and do not have explicit family planning strategies, those who get their contraceptives from other sources, those who practise for longer or shorter periods, those who dislike specific methods or services, those pregnant, those who want to get pregnant, and those who are lost in record systems. Many of these women need services of various and specific kinds; the information that they are 'drop-outs' is neither helpful in this respect, nor accurate.

Discontinuation is not the simple obverse of first method continuation. This definition, while convenient for measurement purposes, ignores variations in number and sequence of methods used and gaps in use. Study of continuation ('acceptors') or discontinuation ('drop-outs') in isolation, either at single points in time or in terms of one contraceptive method, gives a distorted picture of actual contraceptive practice, and neglects the differential development and impact of services.

The situation is further complicated by the negative moral overtones of the way discontinuers are described in the literature. 'Drop-outs' suggests failure on the part of either the user or the programme. This is hardly conducive to understanding the goings-on in other societies, or situations in which service and research personnel are likely to have only partial information.

The term 'drop-out' could probably only come to have explanatory value in the absence of knowledge and awareness of sequential patterns of contraceptive use and disuse. That discontinuers are 'drop-outs' has simply been assumed. In this situation, 'drop-outs' is a convenient guess which roughly circumscribes a poorly understood and poorly differentiated aggregate of people who are seen as a potential problem, or even a threat. As the problem has attained more and more significance, a number of further inferences of the same sort have been added in an attempt to identify broad and simple characteristics of this so-called group: 'motivated' versus 'unmotivated'; 'limiter' versus 'spacer', 'medical' versus 'non-medical' and so forth. These classifications have an ambiguous empirical basis, and have not yielded clear results. Really, they have substituted for a fresh formulation of the problem.

In this respect it may be noted that the predominant research strategies in the area were designed originally for other purposes, and have been further burdened with the task of identifying what are often superficial positive trends in user status. Thus, serious empirical enquiry has tended to be confused with promotional issues. A more realistic picture of patterns of use and discontinuation will very likely be of greater help for both of these purposes, since it must be directed in part to identifying 'drop-outs' who are in fact nothing of the sort.

Critical review of the literatures on use-effectiveness and clinic discontinuation has shown, nonetheless, that the work to date provides a useful foundation. The writings establish the prevalence of first method IUD and pill discontinuation, and also suggest that there are long and short term patterns of continuation. They indicate that many of the women one would expect to want to contracept for age and parity related reasons do in fact try to regulate their fertility. This research indicates widespread dissatisfaction with the methods themselves, especially in connection with physical discomforts. And it suggests that clinics may contribute to these problems, not only by failing to identify and intervene in specific aspects of user-method difficulty, but by adding unnecessary bureaucratic and cultural barriers.

When we turn to the question of what is to be done in order to better understand who and what discontinuation entails, past research has made three further contributions. First it has clarified for the problems of discontinuation the limit of external measurements, and of various calculations based upon them, to provide in themselves the information needed for programme purposes. Specifically, these measures are inappropriate for discerning the presence or absence, and specific content and operation of contraceptive strategies. Nor are they helpful in discerning the motives and practice of that majority of women who contracept but who apparently lack long term strategies of the family planning variety. They are, in addition, unable to cope effectively with the multiplicity of variations in methods used.

Second, existing research and programme operations have led to simple and practiceable record-keeping, survey and experimental evaluation techniques which seem adaptable to certain aspects of the problems of identifying patterns of post-termination events. Third, they have set in motion a wider concern with the contexts in which programmes operate, which emphasizes both improvements in existing operations and interesting alternate channels which may increase the availability, number, and local acceptability of fertility regulating methods.

As a consequence of the way writings have developed

on or around discontinuation, our knowledge of the problem is very uneven. We know much more about some aspects than others, and accordingly, we find research and evaluation techniques unequally developed and employed. It has been possible to hypothesize patterns of use and discontinuation and to point to existing record-keeping systems to help get the needed information. However, the interpretation of the patterns can only avoid the familiar pitfalls and ambiguities of the 'drop-out' variety of inference by actually making the effort to understand local definitions, conditions and processes. In short, the inferences require an empirical base in the cultures and material conditions of the communities in which programmes operate. The outstanding question is the extent to which regular sequences of use and discontinuation can be associated with recurring user problems and experiences. The matching question, if services are to be generally improved and specifically directed to some of these groups of disusers, has to do with staff attitudes and experiences.

A working solution to discontinuation will in any case have to cope with the factors here identified. No single answer to the problem seems possible. The proposition of listing 'reasons' for 'dropping out' thus dissolves into a comparison of local constraints upon users with a record of their interaction with family planning organizations, in the context of general improvements in services. The subsequent courses of action in follow-up of disusers will be decided by organizational practicalities and the possibilities open at the local level.

TABLE I

IUD : Cumulative Discontinuation by months use, First method.

Country; Source;Location	Sample Size	12	24	36	48	Comments
Barbados (201)	-	24.3				Average of several rates reported
Bangladesh						
(275) National	-	26.0	34.0			
Chile						
(201) Santiago	-	15.6	22.7	28.1	32.3	
		26.7	35.5	42.7	47.8	First segment
Colombia (97,200)	-	31.0				
Fiji (201)	-	13.9	23.4			
		24.5	35.7			First segment
Hong Kong						
(45) Territory	1,451	33.9				
India						
(1) New Delhi	867	21.0	36.8			First segment
(275)	-	23.0	46.0			
(236) New Delhi	2,000	49.7	62.7	73.0	80.7	
(167,221) 19 Urban Centres	19,306	22.3	44.0			
Indonesia						
(322) Mojokerto, Java	878	15.0	25.0			
(227) East Java	1,521	13.2	21.2			
(7) Bali	1,824	10.0				
International Post-partum Programme (306)	4,700	21.7	34.8	45.3	54.3	
Iran						
(287) Shiraz	641	19.7	30.4			First segment
Korea						
(153) National 1966	2,184	38.6				
National 1967	2,427	43.4	62.3	74.8		
(14) Koyang	2,283	33.2	52.0			First segment
(172) Seoul	9,207	44.5	62.7	76.5		
Sungbuk Gu	209	51.6				To 12th cycle
(390) Koyang	431	59.0				First segment
Malaysia, West						
(275, 306)	-	32.0	48.0			
Mauritius						
(389) National	-	32.3				
Mexico						
(142) Mexico City	5,381	36.0	60.0			
Morocco						
(216) National	553	28.7	44.7			
Pakistan						
(104) National	1,731	44.2				
(201,265) Lulliani	1,162	37.1	69.4			First segment
Peru						
(200) Lima	-	66.0				

Table I

Country; Source; Location	Sample Size	12	24	36	48	Comments
Philippines						
(183) 'Christian Areas'	-	23.2	37.0			Uncited number of IUDs out of a several method sample of 1,865.
El Salvador						
(200) National	-	37.0	57.0			
Singapore (382)	5,288	31.2				
Sri Lanka						
(275,306)	300	19.0	31.0			
(388)	291	20.0	32.0			
Taiwan						
(250) Taichung	7,295	34.4	51.3			First segment
(90) National, 1966	4,648	37.8	56.7			First segment
		33.1	48.9			
(61) National, 1968	4,972	40.1	57.0	68.3	76.7	First segment
		33.3	47.0	56.9	64.0	
Thailand						
(369) Potharam	902	30.1	43.7	53.3	58.7	
(315) Bangkok	-	14.8	28.7	43.3		
(366,275)	700	24.0	44.0			
Tunisia						
(360) National	1,136	25.4	41.5	53.3	61.7	First segment
		20.5	32.9	42.8	52.2	
Turkey						
(275,362) National	-	38.0				
USA						
(309) Navajo	543	28.0	49.0	60.0		
(191)	6,733		40.5			First segment
(353) Cooperative statistical program	9,974	22.6	34.4	43.4	50.1	Results for Loop D.

Numbers in parenthesis refer to bibliographic citations.
Dashes indicate that the original source was not available at the time of writing, or that the compilation from which rates were drawn did not indicate the relevant information.

TABLE II

Oral Contraceptives : Cumulative discontinuation by months use, First method.

Country;Source;Location	Sample Size	12	24	36	48	Comments
Bangladesh (143)	1,180	88.0				Twelve cycles
Colombia (97,200)	-	53.0				
Haiti (130,240)	149	39.6				Abbreviated Tietze/ Lewit Formula
Hong Kong						
(45) National	1,451	41.8				
India						
(211) Urban Centres	1,512	60.7				
(207) 144 National clinics	9,387	40.5				The pill was provided to women unable to accept the IUD.
(32) Bombay	420	52.9				
(130) Bombay	324	46.9	51.4	58.5	66.0	
	649	28.9	44.8	70.1		
(197) Howrah	609	38.9				Samples refer to geographical areas, respectively urban, rural, slums; to twelfth cycle.
	418	33.4				
	474	69.4				
Indonesia						
(7) Bali	369	40.0				
(227) East Java	1,706	46.5	62.2			
(322) Mojokerto, Java	729	41.0	56.0			
International Postpartum program (306)	4,700	42.2	64.4	76.0		
Korea						
(53) National	1,149	62.0				First segment
(306) National	-	71.0	84.0			First segment
(188) Kyungpook	549	76.0				First segment
(13) Koyang	-	59.0				
Malaysia, West						
(275, 306)	-	38.0	53.0			
Mauritius						
(389) National	-	46.8				
Mexico						
(142) Mexico City	5,381	50.0	66.0			
Morocco						
(216) National	448	54.9	73.4			
Philippines						
(183) 'Christian areas'	-	46.0	64.7			Uncited number of pill users out of a several method sample of 1,865.
Puerto Rico						
(288) Humacao	562	43.2	62.8	74.5	77.4	
(240) Humacao	243	23.9				Abbreviated Tietze/ Lewit Formula.
(240) San Juan	438	45.4				Abbreviated Tietze/ Lewit Formula.

Table II

Country;Source;Location	Sample Size	12	24	36	48	Comments
Singapore						
(132) National	2,969	46.9				
(370) National	2,969	50.0	62.8			
(371) National	2,373	52.5	65.4	71.1	75.3	
Sri Lanka						
(275,306)	300	65.0				
(130)	651	24.3	44.5	65.2		
(388)	322	60.0	70.0			
Taiwan						
(50) National	2,401	69.0				
Thailand						
(275,366)	700	28.5				Average of rates reported.
(306) 16 Districts	-	31.0	45.0			
Tunisia						
(360)	924	76.0	84.4		92.4	First segment
		68.5	77.8		92.4	First segment

Numbers in parenthesis refer to bibliographic citations.
Dashes indicate that the original source was not available at the time of writing, or that the compilation from which rates were drawn did not indicate the relevant information.

TABLE III

IUD Discontinuation by Reasons : Percentages, First Method.

Country; Source: Location	Sample Size	Duration of study in months	Pregnancy	Expulsion	Removal : Medical or side effects	Removal : Planned Pregnancy	Removal : Personal or other	Method change	LFU	Comments
Hong Kong										
(45) National	1,451	12	2.2	7.2	19.0	1.5	4.0		12.0	
India										
(1) New Delhi	867	12	1.2	7.6	13.2				10.1	First segment
		24	2.8	9.9	27.7					First segment
Indonesia										
Mojokerto										
(322) Java	878	12	2.0	6.0	4.0	1.0	2.0			
		24	2.0	11.0	5.0	3.0	4.0		6.2	% of 100 women-months use.
(227) East Java	1,521	12	2.3			1.1	9.8	4.4		'Removal' includes
		24	3.6			2.9	14.7	6.4		expulsion, method changes.
International										
Postpartum										
Program (306)	4,700	12	2.0	6.9	8.5	0.9	3.1			
		24	3.4	9.8	13.2	2.3	5.2			
		36	3.9	11.8	18.0	4.3	6.1			
		48	4.4	13.6	21.4	5.9	7.7			
Iran										
(287) Shiraz	641	12	1.8	1.8	10.0		6.1		40.6	First segment
		24	3.5	1.8	16.1		9.0		40.0	
Korea										
(153) National 1966	2,184	12	2.0	10.6	26.0					First segment
National 1967	2,427	12	2.9	12.4	28.2					First segment
		24	4.2	16.4	41.7					
		36	4.9	17.9	52.0					
(14) Koyang	2,283	12	3.7	9.4	20.7					First segment
(296) Seoul	9,738	12	1.2-4.1	2.7-7.5	8.0-13.2		3.8-7.7			First segment
(172) Seoul	9,207	12	1.8	8.5	34.2					
		24	3.0	10.0	49.7					
		36	3.8	11.6	61.1				34.9	First segment

TABLE III

Korea										
Sungbuk Gu	209	15	6.4	4.7	89.8			65.0		To fifteenth cycle
Mexico										
(142) Mexico City	5,381	21			14.0		64.0	62.0		
Morocco										
(216) National	553	12	2.3	10.1	14.5	1.1	0.2	13.7	43.6	
		24	4.0	14.3	22.7	2.0	0.8			
		36	5.1	17.2	27.1	2.0	1.2			
		48	6.1	17.2	31.7	2.7	2.1			
Pakistan										
(104) National	1,731	12	0.4	20.9	20.8	0.2	1.0		43.0	Expulsion total represents a sum of several categories
Philippines										
(183) 'Christian areas'	174	24	12.1	26.4	44.3	5.7	11.5		24.4	%of discontinuation
Singapore (382)	5,288	12	2.4	17.5	21.4					
Taiwan										
(245) Taichung	7,295	12	4.5	12.2	15.1		2.6			
		24	8.2	14.9	22.0		6.2			
(90,233)National	4,648	12	7.8	10.1	25.0		2.7			Gross termination rates First segment
(61) National	4,972	12	4.8	8.3	18.8					
		24	7.7	10.2	39.1					
		36	9.0	10.7	48.5					
		48	9.5	11.4	55.9					
Thailand										
(369) Potharam	902	12	0.9	6.6	18.3	1.2	3.1			
		24	1.7	11.6	24.2	2.1	4.1			
		36	3.1	13.9	28.8	2.8	4.7			
		48	3.5	15.6	30.8	3.7	5.1			
(315)Bangkok	-	12	1.6	2.3	8.2	1.9	0.8		40.0	
		24	4.2	3.7	14.4	5.1	1.3			
		36	5.1	6.5	20.9	7.7	3.1			

TABLE III

Tunisia (360) National	1,136	12	3.2	6.6	14.0		3.9	33.6	
		24	4.0	10.5	22.5		6.5		
		36	4.4	10.9	30.9		8.2		
		48	4.8	12.4	34.6		10.2		
USA Cooperative Statistical Program (353) Loop D	9,974	12	2.4	4.8	12.9	0.6	1.9		Results for Loop D.
		24	3.6	6.0	19.5	1.8	3.5		
		36	4.2	6.7	24.6	3.1	4.8		
		48	4.9	7.0	28.0	4.2	6.0		
		60	5.1	7.1	30.2	5.3	6.9		
		72	5.4	7.1	31.3	5.8	7.8		

Percentages are calculated per 100 users unless otherwise noted.

TABLE IV

Oral Contraceptive discontinuation by Reasons : Percentages, First method

Country; Source;Location	Sample Size	Duration of study in months	Pregnancy	Planning Pregnancy	Medical or side effects	Personal or other	Method change	LFU	Comments
Haiti									
(130,240)	149	12	7.0			23.8			Abbreviated Tietze/ Lewit Formula, pregnancies and side effects
Hong Kong (45)	1,451	12	2.3	4.5	8.2	9.4	15.6	12.0	
India									
(211) urban areas	1,512	12		10.4	35.1	25.6			
(282) 4 southern states	2,749	36	3.9	6.4	10.0	20.1	1.5	39.3	
(207) 144 National clinics clinics	9,387	12	4.6	4.6	41.3	40.4	1.5	20.7	% of discontinuation; preg. & planning preg. listed together; method change includes only sterilization.
Indonesia									
(322) Majokerto, Java	729	12	6.0	4.0	15.0	17.0			
		24	8.0	6.6	19.0	24.0		9.3	
(227) East Java	1,706	12	4.0	5.8		24.4	11.1		'other' includes medical
		24	5.3	8.0		31.3	15.9		
International Postpartum Program (306)	4,700	12	1.8	3.9	17.8	19.6			
		24	3.6	6.1	26.6	24.1			
		36	3.6	8.0	31.8	27.9			
Korea									
(188) Kyungpook	451	12	2.7	9.0	49.4	37.2	1.7		% of discontinuation, first segment.
(13) Koyang	-	12	0.5	12.2	27.4	29.2	1.0	4.7	
Mexico									
(142) Mexico City	5,381	21			32.0	31.0	22.0		
Morocco									
(216) National	448	12	6.9	3.8	33.7	10.5	9.1	41.1	
		24	9.1	4.8	45.1	14.4			
		36	10.7	5.5	52.8	14.9			

TABLE IV

Philippines									
(183) 'Christian areas'	588	24	6.5	4.9	65.8	22.8			% of discontinuation
Puerto Rico									
(286) San Juan	438	12	18.1			18.7			
(130,240) Humacao	243	12	10.2			6.0			
(288) Humacao	562	12	18.4			11.4		4.1	Duration by number of cycles
		24	16.7			8.6		3.3	
		36	15.0			8.0		3.5	
Singapore									
(132) National	2,969	18	11.0		22.0	10.0		33.0	% of discontinuation; preg., planning preg. combined.
(370) National	1,821	30	9.0		25.0	66.0			
(371) National	2,373	60	22.0		25.0	24.0	17.0	9.0	
Taiwan									
(50) National	2,401	12	1.0		49.8	17.8		8.0	
Tunisia									
(360) National	924	12	3.5	5.9	36.4	9.6	23.7		
		24	5.1	7.0	48.5	12.8			
		36	5.3	7.9	54.6	15.0			
		48	6.5	9.6	57.4	17.5			

Percentages are calculated per 100 users unless otherwise noted.

TABLE V

Method Changes

Country; Source; Location	Duration in months	First Method	Continuation rate	Restart	Discontinuation	Method Change	IUD	Pill	Sterilized	Other	Abortion	Drop-out	Comments
India													
(236) New Delhi	48	IUD	19.3	4.0	80.7	52.4			21.4	31.0		33.7	Changes are by % of terminators
(1)	24	IUD	63.2	21.0	36.8	14.0						5.0	
Korea													
(390) Seoul	12	IUD-Pill	41.0	11.0	59.0	39.0						35.7	Special offer of pills to IUD drop-outs. Changes are by % of terminators.
			55.3		44.7			86.1					
Morocco													
(216) National	24	IUD	34.0		66.0		50.0			18.3			%of terminators changing from pill to IUD or vice versa.
Philippines													
(183) 'Christian areas'	24	IUD Pill	73.1 50.2				15.0	24.0		Rhythm 23 With-drawal 24 Other 14			All-method continuation rates; changes are by % of terminators
Singapore													
(132) National	12	Pill	53.1	3.5	46.9	65.0							Changes are by %of terminators.
Taiwan													
(90) Island wide	30	IUD	53.6	7.7	38.7	14.2					9.0	24.5	
(90) Taichung	53	IUD	47.4	7.9	44.7	17.7					4.0	27.0	
(125) Island wide	12	Pill	41.0	15.0	59.0		8.0			10.0		44.0	
Tunisia													
(360) National	48		38.3		61.7			15.3		18.3		66.5	Continuation by First segment Change data by %of terminators by method.
	48		7.6		92.4		5.5			18.2		76.0	
Trinidad-Tobago													
(102)	6	Pill	44.0			22.0						34.0	

Continuation data calculated by first method rates.
Method change data is by % of sample, unless otherwise noted.

Bibliographical Note

The bibliography is compiled almost entirely on the basis of resources available in the IPPF Central Office Library. It covers published and unpublished materials related to discontinuation in Asia, Africa and Latin America for the period 1966-1976. Most of these fall into the period 1971-1976. The great majority of the material is in English, although a few articles in French and Spanish are included.

Although the literature specific to drop-outs is small, the related materials are copious. The problem in compiling the bibliography has been to select the more helpful articles on a topic which cuts across four related but diverse family planning methodologies: 1. studies directed to KAP-type variables; 2. research on the use-effectiveness of specific contraceptives; 3. problems in clinic management and record-keeping; and 4. studies of cultural and psychological aspects of method and clinic discontinuation. There is an obvious artificiality to these distinctions. For example, a paper on clinic waiting times or a tabulation of drop-outs by age, education, etc. will not overlap a discussion of births-averted; but writings on postpartum family planning may take in them all.

Of the four areas only the first receives scant attention, in part because it comprises an immense literature in its own right, and in part because it does not contain the longitudinal information needed to assess continuing patterns of use and discontinuation. The bulk of the bibliography is made up of materials falling in the second category, since discussion of discontinuation and 'drop-outs' almost inevitably reflects use-effectiveness measures. Indeed papers included in the third and fourth categories usually only offer variations on this methodology, as I have tried to indicate in the text. It is impossible to give precise percentages of coverage since the literature relevant to the topic has no simple boundaries, and many unpublished papers may have eluded my attention. The bibliography represents in my guess at least 75% of materials in English as of mid-1976.

An addendum of 10 items has been included to cover principal publications related to the topic during the months in which the manuscript was being revised. These writings do not seem to have changed the situation described in the text.

It is worth noting that two recent papers develop criticisms of the life table method of measuring discontinuation, one from a mathematical viewpoint (401), the other (399) in terms of improving the technique according to its original purpose in this field, viz. assessing the performance of the IUD in clinical trials. Thus neither article is addressed to the inadequacy of the method as it is currently used as an evaluative measure of social programme performance.

BIBLIOGRAPHY

1 AGARWALA, S.N. India

1968 A follow-up study of intrauterine contraceptive devices: an Indian experience. Eugenics Quarterly, 15, 1, 41-49.

2 AGER, J.W. U.S.A.

1973 Correlates of continuance in a family planning program. Journal of Obstetric, Gynecologic and Neonatal Nursing, 2, 15-23.

3 ALERS, J.O. Thailand

1971 ... C. SUVANAVEJH: Continuation of contraceptive practice in Thailand: the 1971 follow-up survey. Population Council Quarterly Reports, Thailand. Pp. 13.

4 ALI, N.H. Bangladesh

1971 A study of family planning drop-outs. In: Two studies in family planning. Comilla: East Pakistan Academy for Rural Development. Pp. 34.

5 AMAL, S.H. Indonesia

1975 Motivation and continuation of family planning acceptors in Ketamatan Serpong, West Java. Family Planning Project, Serpong, Indonesia, Leyden State University. Serpong Paper No. 11 Pp. 37.

6 APELO, R.A. Philippines
1974 ... J.R. DE LA CRUZ, F.C. LOPEZ: Acceptability of injectable contraception in the Philippines. IPPF Medical Bulletin, 8, 2, 1-2.

7 ASTAWA, I.B. Indonesia
1975 ... S. WALOEYO, J.E. LAING: Family planning in Bali. Studies in Family Planning, 6, 4, 86-101.

8 AVERY, R.C. Taiwan
1973 Patterns and implications of long-term IUD use in Taichung, Taiwan. Studies in Family Planning, 4, 6, 139-143.

9 BAILEY, J. Colombia
1975 ... J. CORREA: Evaluation of the profamilia rural family planning program. Studies in Family Planning, 6, 6, 148-155.

10 BALLWEG, J.A. Philippines
1974 ... D.W. MACCORQUODALE: Family planning method change and drop-outs in the Philippines. Social Biology, 21, 1, 88-95

11 BAMBERGER, M. Venezuela
1971 ... M. EARLE: Factors affecting the success of a family planning programme in a low-income neighbourhood in Caracas. Studies in Family Planning, 2, 8, 175-178.

12 BANG, S. Korea
1966 The Koyang study: results of two action programs. Studies in Family Planning, 1, 11, 5-12.

13 1968 ... S.W. SONG, B.B. YOUN: Field study of an oral contraceptive among IUD drop-outs in rural Korea. Yonsei Medical Journal, 9, 2, 168-184.

14 1968 ... S.W. SONG, C.H. CHOI: Improving access to the IUD: experiments in Koyang, Korea. Studies in Family Planning, 1, 27, 4-11.

15 1970 Can IUD retention be improved by prompt check-up visits? In: Population and Family Planning in the Republic of Korea, Vol. 1. Ministry of Health and Social Affairs, Republic of Korea, Pp. 130-135.

16 1971 Korea: The relationship between IUD retention and check-up visits. Studies in Family Planning, 2, 5, 110-112.

17 BANHARNSUPAWAT, L. Thailand

1971 ... A.G. ROSENFIELD: Immediate post-partum IUD insertions. Obstetrics and Gynaecology, 38, 2, 276-285.

18 BARDWICK, J.M. Various

1973 Psychological factors in the acceptance and use of oral contraceptives. In: Psychological Perspectives on Population, J.M. Fawcett (ed.) Pp. 274-305.

19 BARGLOW, P. U.S.A.

1972 ... D. KLASS: Psychiatric aspects of contraceptive utilization. American Journal of Obstetrics and Gynecology, 114, 1, 93-6.

20 BARRON, B.A. Barbados
1969 ... H. WEINSTEIN, R.M. RICHART: An investigation of the effects of the intrauterine contraceptive device based on a longitudinal study of a self-selected sample of Barbadian women. American Journal of Obstetrics and Gynecology, *124*, 7, 723-729.

21 BAUMAN, K.E. Thailand
1972 ... P. VARAJEV: Reason for contracepting and choice between IUD and pill: implications for the difference in continuation rates. Social Biology, *19*, 3, 292-296.

22 BEASLEY, J.D. U.S.A.
1970 ... R.F. FRANKOWSKI. Utilization of a family planning program by the poor population of a metropolitan area. Milbank Memorial Fund Quarterly, *48*, 241-281.

23 1971 ... R.F. FRANKOWSKI, C.M. HAWKINS: Louisiana family planning. American Journal of Public Health, *61*, 9, 1812-1825.

24 BELSKY, R. Various
1975 Barrier methods: vaginal contraceptives; a time for reappraisal? Population Reports, *3*, 37-56.

25 BERELSON, B. Various
1969 National family planning programs: where we stand. Studies in Family Planning, *1*, 39, 341-387.

26 BERGGREN, G.G. Haiti
1974 ... H.W. VAILLANT, N. GARNIER: Lippes loop insertion by mid-wives in healthy and chronically ill women in rural Haiti. American Journal of Public Health, 64, 7, 719-22.

27 BERNARD, R.P. Various
1970 IUD performance patterns: a 1970 world view. International Journal Gynaecology and Obstetrics, 8, 6, (pt. 2), 926-940.

28 1971 Factors governing IUD performance. American Journal of Public Health 61, 3, 559-567.

29 1972 The "M"-IUD: an international clinical trial. American Journal of Public Health, 62, 6, 828-845.

30 BERTERA, R.L. Various
1973 Population/family planning programs annotated bibliography of evaluation methodologies. Technical Information Service: Carolina Population Center, University of North Carolina, Bibliography Series, Number 5, Pp. 18.

31 BHATHENA, R.K. India
1971 ... S.D. KANITKAR: Analysis of 'drop-outs' in oral contraceptives. Current Medical Practice, 15, 10, 972-975.

32 BHENDE, A. India
1969 ... D.N. SAKSENA: A study of oral contraceptive users in Bombay. Bombay: International Institute for Population Studies. Pp. 36.

33 BOGUE, D.J. Various
1971 ... J. NELSON: The fertility components and contraceptive techniques for measuring contraceptive use-effectiveness. Community and Family Study Center. University of Chicago. Evaluation Manual 5. Pp. 75.

34 BORLAND, B.L. Various
1972 Behavioural factors in non-coital methods of contraception: a review. Social Sciences and Medicine, 6, 1, 163-78.

35 BRACKEN, N.B. Jamaica
1973 ... S.V. KASL: Factors associated with dropping out of family planning clinics in Jamaica. American Journal of Public Health, 63, 3, 262-271.

36 1976 Contraception and pregnancy after dropping out of family planning clinics: a national interview survey in Jamaica. Social Biology, 23, 1, 55-65.

37 BRADSHAW, R. U.S.A.
1972 ... F. PERAGALLO: Contraceptive discontinuation among patients using oral and intrauterine methods. In: Advances in Planned Parenthood, Vol. 7. Proceedings, Ninth Annual Meeting of the American Association for Planned Parenthood Physicians, Kansas City, Missouri, April 5-6, 1971. A.J. Sobrero, R.M. Harvey (eds.). Amsterdam: Excerpta Medica. Pp. 42-55.

38 BRODY, E.B. Jamaica
1974 Psychocultural aspects of contraceptive behaviour in Jamaica. Journal of Nervous and Mental Disease, 159, 2, 108-119.

39 BUMPASS, L. U.S.A.
1970 ... C.F. WESTOFF: The later years of childbearing. Pp. 168.

40 CASTADOT, R.G. Various
1975 ... et al.: The International Post-Partum Family Planning Program: Eight years of experience. Reports on Population/Family Planning, 18, Pp. 53.

41 CENTRO DE INVESTIGACIONES SOCIALES POR MUESTREO Peru
1969 Evaluación de programas de planificación familiar. Lima: Ministerio de Trabajo.

42 CERNADA, G.P. Taiwan
1970 ... T.H. SUN: Recent findings: an inventory. In: Taiwan Family Planning Reader: How a Program Works. G. Cernada (ed.) Pp. 281-292.

43 1972 ... L.P. LU: The Kaoshiung study. Studies in Family Planning, 3, 8, 198-203.

44 1973 Family planning drop-outs and how to communicate with them. In: Family Planning Communications in Taiwan Area, Republic of China. The Chinese Center for International Training in Family Planning, Pp. 17.

45 CHAN, K.C. Hong Kong
1971 Hong Kong: oral contraceptive follow-up study. Studies in Family Planning, 2, 3, 70-74.

46 1971 Hong Kong: report of the IUD Reassurance Project. Studies in Family Planning, 2, 11, 225-233.

47 CHANDRASEKARAN, C. Various

1971 ... D.V.R. MURTY, K. SRINIVASAN: Some problems in determining the number of acceptors needed in a family planning programme to achieve a specified reduction in the birth rate. Population Studies, 25, 2, 303-308.

48 1972 ... M. KARKAL: "Continuation rate", "use-effectiveness" and their assessment for the diaphragm and jelly method. Population Studies, 26, 3, 487-494.

49 1975 ... A.I. HERMALIN (eds.). Measuring the effect of family planning programs on fertility. International Union for the Scientific Study of Population. Pp. 570.

50 CHEN, F.L. Taiwan

1970 ... et. al.: Taiwan: first island-wide pill acceptor follow-up survey. Studies in Family Planning, 1, 60, 18-23.

51 CHEN, J.S. Taiwan

1975 ... et al.: IUD reinsertion in Taichung: a study of first and later segments. Studies in Family Planning, 6, 9, 338-44.

52 CHESLER, J. South Africa

1961 The use of contraceptive diaphragms: a follow-up study. South African Medical Journal, 35, 323-4.

53 CHO, K.S. Korea

1970 ... E.S. KIM, E.I. KIM: Study on the acceptability and effectiveness of oral contraceptives among Korean women. National Family Planning Center, Pp. 59. (Korean with English summary).

54 CHOW, L.P. Taiwan

1965 A programme to control fertility in Taiwan: setting, accomplishment and evaluation. Population Studies, 19, 2, 155-166.

55 1965 ... H.C. CHEN, T.T. RUANG, T.C. HSU, Evaluation of an IUD program by follow-up interview. Formosan Medical Association, 64, 7, 345-357.

56 1967 ... R. FREEDMAN: Taiwan: births averted by the IUD program. Studies in Family Planning, 1, 20, 7-8.

57 1968 ... R. FREEDMAN, R.G. POTTER, A.K. JAIN: Correlates of IUD termination in a mass family planning program: the first Taiwan IUD follow-up survey. Milbank Memorial Fund Quarterly, 46, 2 pt. 1, 215-236.

58 1968 Evaluation of the family planning program in Taiwan, Republic of China. Formosan Medical Association, 67, 7, 280-307.

59 1970 Family Planning in Taiwan, Republic of China: progress and prospects. Population Studies, 24, 3, 339-352.

60 1970 Role of the IUD in a national family planning program. International Journal of Gynaecology and Obstetrics, 8, 5, 2 pt., 698-708.

61 1974 The island-wide family planning program in Taiwan: analysis of accomplishments of the past eight years. Population Studies, 28, 1, 107-126.

62 CHUNG, B.M. Korea
1972 ... J.A. PALMORE, S.J. LEE: Psychological perspectives in family planning in Korea. Korean Institute for Research in the Behavioural Sciences, Pp. 532.

63 CHUNG, C.S. Korea
1972 ... S.J. YU: Evaluation of a study in acceptance and continuation of oral contraceptives among women in a rural area. In: Sociological Evaluation of the Family Planning Programs and Research Activities in Korea. Korean Sociological Association. Pp. 167-182.

64 COBLINER, W.G. U.S.A.
1975 ... H. SCHULMAN, V. SMITH: Patterns of contraceptive failures: the role of motivation re-examined. Journal of Biosocial Science, 7, 3, 307-18.

65 COCHRANE, C.M. U.S.A.
1973 ... et. al.: Motivational determinants of family planning attendance. Journal of Psychology, 84, 33-43.

66 CONCEPCION, M. Philippines
1972 ... C.L. LORENZO, JR: Philippines. Studies in Family Planning, 3, 7, 140-142.

67 CORFMAN, P.A. U.S.A.
1971 A five-year plan for population research and family planning services: 2. Population research. Family Planning Perspectives, 3, 4, 41-48.

68 CROSS, M. Trinidad and Tobago
1976 Family planning in Trinidad and Tobago: the problem of discontinuation. Interim Report to the International Planned Parenthood Federation.

69 DAVIES, P.J. Brazil
1976 ... W. RODRIGUES: Community-based distribution of oral contraceptives in Rio Grande do Norte, Northeastern Brazil. Studies in Family Planning, 7, 7, 202-207.

70 DEMOGRAPHIC ASSOCIATION OF EL SALVADOR El Salvador
n.d Descripción del funcionamiento de servicios de planificación familiar en los Centros Asistenciales del Ministerio de Salud.

71 DHARMAPANIJ, T. Thailand
n.d. ... M.R. SURAVARN VORAVARN, S. PANYARUCHUN: Immediate post-partum IUD insertions, Vajira Hospital, Bangkok. Vajira Medical Journal, Pp. 6.

72 DINGLE, J.T. U.S.A.
1963 ... C. TIETZE: Comparative study of three contraceptive methods: vaginal foam tablets, jelly alone, and diaphragm with jelly or cream. American Journal of Obstetrics and Gynecology, 85, 8, 1012-1021.

73 EAST PAKISTAN RESEARCH AND EVALUATION CENTER — Bangladesh

1968 East Pakistan IUD retention study (preliminary report).

74 EBANKS, G.E. — Barbados

1968 Patterns of contraceptive use among clients of the Barbados Family Planning Association. Unpublished Ph.D. thesis, Cornell University, Pp. 253.

75 1969 Patterns of contraceptive use among clients of the Barbados Family Planning Association. Dissertation Abstracts, <u>29</u>, 11A, 4113.

76 1969 Social and demographic characteristics of family planning clients in Barbados. Social and Economic Studies, <u>18</u>, 391-401.

77 1970 Users and non-users of contraception: tests of stationarity applied to members of a family planning programme. Population Studies, <u>24</u>, 1, 85-91.

78 ECHEVERRY, G. — Colombia

1973 Family Planning in the immediate post-partum period. Studies in Family Planning, <u>4</u>, 2, 33-35.

79 1975 Development of the Profamilia rural family planning program in Colombia. Studies in Family Planning, <u>6</u>, 6, 142-147.

80 EWER, P.A. — U.S.A.

1971 ... J.O. GIBBS: Correlates of oral contraception continuation. Health Services and Mental Health Administration Reports, <u>86</u>, 5, 449-456.

81 FAMILY WELFARE PLANNING PROJECT HUMANITY ASSOCIATION — India

1973 An exploratory study of the effect of oral pills on Indian women: A final review of a project of the Pathfinder Fund. Howrah, India. Pp. 22.

82 FAWCETT, J.T. — Thailand

1967 ... A. SOMBOONSUK, S. KHAISANG: Thailand: an analysis of time and distance factors at an IUD clinic in Bangkok. Studies in Family Planning, 1, 19, 8-12.

83 1969 Thailand: using family planning acceptors to recruit new cases. Studies in Family Planning, 1, 39, 1-4.

84 FEINERMAN, D. — France

1972 ... I. RABARISON, J. COHEN: Enquête de surveillance de femmes sous contraception. Fertilité Orthongénie, 4, 1, 33-44.

85 FELDMAN, J.G. — U.S.A.

1971 ... J. LIPPES: Four-year comparison between the utilization and use-effectiveness of sequential and combined oral contraceptives. Contraception, 3, 2, 53-104.

86 FINCANCIOGLU, N. — Turkey

1969 Turkish IUD retention survey. Pp. 45.

87 FINNIGAN, O.D. Korea
1970 ... S.D. KOO: The use of postcards in recruiting IUD drop-outs to the pill. In: Ministry of Health and Social Affairs, Population and Family Planning in the Republic of Korea, Vol. 1, Pp. 318-322.

88 FORREST, J.E. Various
1971 Postpartum services in family planning: findings to date. Reports on Population/Family Planning, 8, Pp. 15.

89 FREEDMAN, R. Taiwan
1969 ... T.H. SUN: Who has the IUD reinserted after a first termination? In: Family Planning in Taiwan: An Experiment in Social Change. R. Freedman, J.T. Takeshita (eds.) Pp. 458-484.

90 1969 ... et. al.: The family planning program for all Taiwan. In: Family Planning in Taiwan, R. Freedman, J.T. Takeshita (eds.) Pp. 313-350.

91 1970 ... A.K. JAIN, A.I. HERMALIN, T.H. SUN: Fertility after insertion of an intrauterine device in Taiwan's family planning program. Taiwan Population Studies Working Paper, Number 6, Pp. 20.

92 1970 ... A.K. JAIN, T.H. SUN: Correlates of family limitation in Taiwan after IUD insertion. In: Taiwan Family Planning Reader: How a Program Works. G. Cernada (ed.) Pp. 293-313.

93 1976 ... B. BERELSON: The record of family planning programs. Studies in Family Planning, 7, 1, 1-40. Various

94 FRIEDMAN, H.L. U.S.A.
1973 ... R.L. JOHNSON, E.P. MCCORMICK, H.P. DAVID: Management general service studies of user/system interaction: a prospectus for research. Washington, D.C.: Transnational Family Research Institute. Pp. 10.

95 GILLESPIE, R. Various
1972 Reactions to break-through bleeding with IUD's and orals. Paper for WHO Task Force on Contraceptive Acceptability. Pp. 9.

96 GLUCKMAN, L.K. New Zealand
1969 Psychiatric aspects of failures with oral contraceptives. New Zealand Medical Journal 70, 10-13.

97 GOMEZ, F. Colombia
1972 Abandono al servicio clínico en un programa de planificación familiar en Colombia. Ithaca, NY.: Cornell University. Masters Thesis.

98 GRINBLAT, J.A. Tunisia
1971 Analysis of continuation of pill use from medical records. In: The first African Population Conference, Accra, Ghana. Dec. 9. 1971. U.N. Economic Commission for Africa; International Union for the Scientific Study of Population; the International Planned Parenthood Federation, Accra, Ghana. Pp. 11.

99 GUTIERREZ, H.F. Various
1974 Contraceptive service statistics: basic concepts. International Planned Parenthood Federation, Western Hemisphere Region. Pp. 112.

100 HALL, F. U.S.A.
1969 ... W.A. REINKE: Factors influencing contraception continuation rates: the oral and intrauterine methods. Demography, 6, 3, 335-346.

101 HALL, R. U.S.A.
1973 Continuation and pregnancy rates with four contraceptive methods. American Journal of Obstetrics and Gynecology 116, 5, 671-681.

102 HAREWOOD, J. Trinidad and Tobago
1973 Changes in the use of birth control methods. Population Studies, 27, 1, 33-57.

103 HARTFIELD V.J. Nigeria
1971 The role of the nurse in a family planning programme. Contraception, 3, 2, 105-114.

104 HELBIG, D.W. Pakistan
1970 ... et. al.: IUD retention in West Pakistan and methodology of assessment. Demography, 7, 4, 467-482.

105 HEMACHUDHA, C. Thailand
1972 ... et. al.: Thailand. Studies in Family Planning, 3, 7, 150-156.

106 HERMALIN, A.I. Taiwan
1970 ... L.P. CHOW: Motivational factors in IUD termination: data from the second Taiwan IUD follow-up survey. Ann Arbor: Population Studies Center, University of Michigan. Taichung: Taiwan Provincial Institute of Family Planning. Taiwan Population Studies Working Paper 9.

107 1971 ... L.P. CHOW: Motivational correlates of termination: data from the second Taiwan IUD follow-up survey. Journal of Biosocial Science, 3, 4, 351-375.

108 HERSON, J. Various
1975 Standardization of cumulative failure rates. Demography, 12, 3, 467-470.

109 HILTON, E.T. Various
1975 ... A.A. LUMSDAINE: Field trial designs in gauging the impact of fertility planning programs. In: C.A. Bennett, A.A. Lumsdaine (eds.), Evaluation and Experiment: Some Critical Issues in Assessing Social Programs. Pp. 319-408.

110 HONG KONG: FAMILY PLANNING ASSOCIATION Hong Kong
1970 9th Annual Report, 1969-1970. Pp. 37 (English). Pp. 18 (Chinese).

111 HOSSAIN, M. Bangladesh
1972 Oral contraceptive study. Bangladesh Family Welfare Association. Pp. 59.

112 HSU, T.C. Taiwan

1964 ... L.P. CHOW, S.M. KEENY: The program for intrauterine contraceptive devices in Taiwan: development, setting and evaluation. In: Proceedings of the Second International Conference on Intrauterine Contraception.

113 1964 ... C.H. LEE, C.L. CHOW, L.P. CHOW: Preliminary report and medical follow-up study of new intrauterine contraceptive devices. Journal of the Formosan Medical Association, 63, 9, 427-436.

114 HUBER, S.C. Various

1975 ... et. al.: Contraceptive distribution: taking supplies to villages and households. Population Reports, Series J, Number 5. Department of Medical and Public Affairs, The George Washington University Medical Center, Washington, D.C. Pp. 19.

115 INDONESIA: NATIONAL FAMILY PLANNING BOARD OF DJAKARTA Indonesia

1970 A study concerning the retention rates of early IUD acceptors as part of the post-partum program in Sawah Besar Maternity Clinic. Pp. 11.

116 INDONESIA: THE DCI DJAKARTA FAMILY PLANNING PROJECT

1969 Survey on pill continuance. Pp. 5.

117 1969 IUD retention survey. Pp. 5.

118 INDRAYAN, A. India
1972 ... S.C. BAGCHI, V. VERMA: Medico-social factors contributory to drop-outs in a rural cohort of oral contraceptors. Journal of Family Welfare 18, 4, 65-75.

119 INTERNATIONAL COMMITTEE ON APPLIED RESEARCH IN POPULATION Various
1974 ... (Prepared by E.M. WHELAN): Compliance with contraceptive regimens. Studies in Family Planning, 5, 11, 349-355.

120 1975 ... (Prepared by E.M. WHELAN): Attitudes toward menstruation. Studies in Family Planning, 6, 4, 106-8.

121 INTERNATIONAL IUD PROGRAMME Various
1969 IUD performance patterns. 2 Vols. Boston: Pathfinder Fund.

122 JAFFNA, S.H.S. Sri Lanka
1969 Loop follow-up survey. Family Planning Evaluation Unit, Report number 2. Pp. 6.

123 JAIN, A.K. Taiwan
1969 Relative fecundability of users and non-users of contraception. Social Biology, 16, 1, 39-43.

124 1970 Highlights of the third island-wide follow-up survey of IUD acceptors, 1968. Pp. 3.

125 1974 Relative effectiveness of different fertility control methods in reducing community reproduction rate. In: International Population Conference, Liege, 1973. Vol. 2. International Union for the Scientific Study of Population. Pp. 209-224. — Various

126 JAIN, S.P. — India
1970 On Tietze's method of analysing IUD experience. Journal of Family Welfare, 17, 1, 58-68.

127 JALNAWALLA, S.F. — India
1972 Oral pill project in India. Journal of the Indian Medical Association, 59, 8, 344-8.

128 JARAMILLO-GOMEZ, M. — Ecuador
1972 Report on clinical activities of the Association for the Welfare of the Ecuadorian Family in 1971. Paper prepared for the Association, Pp. 17.

129 JOHNSON, J.T. — Malaysia
1974 Multiple acceptors; a study of repetitive recording of clients as new acceptors in the Malaysian family planning program. Working Paper Number 12, Ann Arbor: University of Michigan, Department of Population Planning, Pp. 46.

130 JONES, G.W. Various
1967 ... W.P. MAUDLIN: Use of oral contraceptives with special reference to developing countries. Studies in Family Planning, 1, 24, 1-13.

131 JOSHI, S.B.R. India
1968 ... K.T. CHITRE: A Survey of condom users. Journal of Family Welfare, 15, 2, 14-22.

132 KANAGARATNAM, K. Singapore
1969 ... K.C. KIM: Singapore: The use of oral contraceptives in the national program. Studies in Family Planning, 1, 48, 1-9.

133 KANE, F.J. Various
1968 Psychiatric reactions to oral contraceptives. American Journal of Obstetrics and Gynecology, 102, 7, 1053-1063.

134 KANITKAR, S.D. India
1972 Bhivpuri family planning project: a well participated rural 'pill' programme. In: Proceedings of the International Conference on Family Planning, New Delhi, March 12-16, 1972, P.C. Bhatla (ed.). Indian Medical Association.

135 KANTNER, J.F. Pakistan
1964 Pakistan: the medical school research project at Lulliani. Studies in Family Planning, 1, 4, 5-9.

136 KARKAL, S.M. — India

1971 Soonawala IUD-SIUD: Experience of women in Bombay. Journal of Family Welfare, 17, 4, 27-37.

137 KEENY, S.M. — Korea Taiwan

1967 Korea and Taiwan: the score for 1966. Studies in Family Planning, 1, 19, 1-7.

138 1968 ... G. CERNADA, J.A. ROSS: Korea and Taiwan: The record for 1967. Studies in Family Planning, 1, 29, 1-9.

139 1970 ... G.P. CERNADA: Taiwan 1969: Report on the national family planning program. Studies in Family Planning, 1, 54, 8-13. — Taiwan

140 1972 East Asia Review. Studies in Family Planning, 3, 7, 125-164. — Various

141 KELLER, A. — Mexico

1971 Mexico City: a clinic drop-out study. Studies in Family Planning, 2, 9, 192-196.

142 1973 Patient attrition in five Mexico City family planning clinics. In: J.M. Stycos (ed.) Clinics, Contraception and Communication. Pp. 25-50.

143 1974 ... A.R. DE RODRIGUEZ, S. CORREU: The Mexican experience with postpartum/postabortion programs, 1970-1972. Studies in Family Planning, 5, 6, 195-200.

144 1975 ... et. al.: The impact of organization of family planning clinics on waiting time. Studies in Family Planning, 6, 5 134-140.

145 KELLY, W.J. Various
1971 Estimation of births averted by family planning programs: the parity approach. Studies in Family Planning, 2, 9, 197-201.

146 1971 Estimation of contraceptive continuation functions. Demography, 8, 3, 335-339.

147 KHAN, A.R. Bangladesh
1975 ... A.F.M. BURHANUDDIN, S.M. D'SOUZA, L.C. CHEN: A study of oral pill acceptors in the Bangladesh postpartum family planning program. Bangladesh Development Studies, 3, 1, 53-76.

148 KIM, C.H. Korea
1973 ... S.J. LEE: Socio-demographic and psychological characteristics of the women using both induced abortion and contraception. Psychological studies in population/family planning, 1, 3. Korean Institute for Research in the Behavioural Sciences.

149 1973 Socio-psychological characteristics of induced abortion repeaters. Psychological studies in population/family planning, 1, 2. Korean Institute for Research in the Behavioural Sciences.

150 KIM, E.I. Korea
1974 ... N.H. CHO, S.H. PARK: A follow-up survey on condom users under the national family planning program. Korean Institute for Research in the Behavioural Sciences. Pp. 77. (In Korean, with English summary).

151 KIM, S.K. Korea
1975 ... Y.H. YANG, S.H. CHUNG: A comparative study on the effectiveness of the Copper-T 200 and Lippes loop in a rural community. Journal of Family Planning Studies, 2, 51-63 (Korean, summary and charts in English).

152 KIM, T.I. Korea
1972 ... et. al.: The Korean national family planning program: population control and fertility decline. New York: Population Council, Pp. 240.

153 KIM, T.R. Korea
1970 National intrauterine contraception report. Seoul: The National Family Planning Centre. Pp. 188.

154 1972 Outline of evaluation research activities for Korea's national family planning program: achievements and problems. In: Sociological Evaluation of the Family Planning Programs and Research Activities in Korea. Seoul: Korean Sociological Association. Pp. 53-82.

155 KOH, Y.B. Korea
1972 ... D.W. KIM: A sociological evaluation of the family planning action programs in rural Korea. In: Sociological Evaluation of the Family Planning Programs and Research Activities in Korea. Seoul: Korean Sociological Association. Pp. 137-147

156 KOHLI, K.L. India
1975 Factors leading to drop-outs among men registered for vasectomy. Journal of Family Welfare, 21, 3, 30-37.

157 KOREAN INSTITUTE FOR FAMILY PLANNING Korea
1971 Korean family planning program in charts, 3rd edition National Family Planning Center. Pp. 38.

158 1974 Korean family planning program in charts, 5th edition National Family Planning Center. Pp. 40.

159 1974 Korean population and family planning bibliography, Pp. 68.

160 1974 Population and family planning in the Republic of Korea. Vol. 2. Pp. 587.

161 KOREA, REPUBLIC OF: MINISTRY OF HEALTH AND SOCIAL AFFAIRS Korea
1966 National intrauterine contraception report. Pp. 133. (Korean and English).

162 1967 National intrauterine contraception report.

163 1970 Findings on status subsequent to insertion of intrauterine contraceptive devices for acceptors in 1964 and 1965 combined. In: Population and Family Planning in the Republic of Korea. Pp. 108-119.

164 1970 Population and family planning in the Republic of Korea, Vol. 1, Pp. 550.

165 KOREA: SCHOOL OF PUBLIC HEALTH, SEOUL NATIONAL UNIVERSITY Korea
1965 Progress report: Sungdong Gu Action Research Project, Part I, Major findings from progress data.

166 KULKARNI, P.N. Taiwan
1976 ... R.G. POTTER, JR.: Extrapolation of IUD continuation curves. Population Studies, 30, 2, 353-368.

167 KUMAR, A. India
1971 An overview of IUCD studies in India. International Institute for Population Studies, Bombay, Pp. 11.

168 KWON, E.R. Korea
1968 ... T.R. KIM, J.J. PARK, K.W. KANG: A study in acceptability and effectiveness of oral pills with women residents in an urban area: based on a program directed towards women having discontinued use of intrauterine contraceptive loops in Sungdong Gu, Seoul, Korea. Journal of Population Studies, 6, 3-139. (Korean and English).

169 1969 ... et. al.: A study of the acceptability and effectiveness of intrauterine contraception in relation to socio-medical variables. Journal of Population Studies, 8.

170 1971 ... et. al.: Some fact findings on pregnancy and birth interval: based on pregnancy history data of currently pregnant women residing in Sungdong Gu, Seoul. Journal of Population Studies, 13, 152-154.

171 1971 ... et. al.: A study on use-effectiveness and extended use-effectiveness of contraceptive methods. Journal of Population Studies 12, 85-107. (In Korean).

172 1972 Study on urban population control. In: Sociological Evaluation of the Family Planning Programme and Research Activities in Korea. Seoul: Korean Sociological Association. Pp. 183-214.

173 1974 Ten years of urban population studies in Korea. Seoul College of Medicine. Pp. 187.

174 KWON, H.Y. Korea
1969 ... J.K. CHAN, D.P. SMITH: Results of the April 1969 IUD resurvey. Family Planning Evaluation Team. Seoul: Ministry of Health and Social Affairs.

175 1972 Some correlates of IUD termination in Korea: an application of the elaboration model for the analysis of correlates on IUD termination rates. Korean Institute for Family Planning. Family Planning Quarterly 3, 87-107.

176 LAING, J.E. Philippines

1971 Continuation and pregnancy rates among acceptors at rhythm clinics in Manila. Population Institute, University of the Philippines, Family Planning Evaluation Center. Pp. 6.

177 1972 Use-effectiveness of family planning in the Philippines, 1970-2. Population Institute, University of the Philippines. Family Planning Evaluation Office. Pp. 26.

178 1973 Differentials in Philippines contraceptive continuation and pregnancy rates. Population Institute, University of the Philippines. Family Planning Evaluation Office. Pp. 29.

179 1973 Family planning clinic density and the acceptance rate: evidence from the Philippines. Population Institute, University of the Philippines, Family Planning Evaluation Office. Pp. 30.

180 1973 Final Report: Recommendations for the program as a whole and for research and evaluation in particular. Population Institute, University of the Philippines, Family Planning Evaluation Center. Pp. 24.

181 1973 Research for management of population program. Population Institute, University of the Philippines. Family Planning Evaluation Center. Pp. 22.

182 1973 Selected response distributions from the 1972 National Acceptor Survey. Population Institute, University of the Philippines, Family Planning Evaluation Office. Pp. 35.

183 1974 Differentials in contraceptive use-effectiveness in the Philippines. Studies in Family Planning, _5_, 10, 302-13.

184 LAPHAM, R.J. Various
1972 ... W.P. MAULDIN: National family planning programmes: review and evaluation. Studies in Family Planning, _3_, 3, 29-52.

185 LECOMTE, J. Morocco, Tunisia
1976 ... A. MARCOUX: Contraception and fertility in Morocco and Tunisia. Studies in Family Planning, _7_, 7, 182-187.

186 LEE, S.K. Korea

1969 ... D.W. HAN, M.H. YE: A study in acceptance and continuation of oral contraceptives among women in a rural area. Korean Journal of Preventive Medicine, 2, 1.

187 1970 ... et. al.: A comparison of side-effects for various kinds of oral contraceptive pills. Korean Journal of Preventive Medicine, 3, 1, 51-95.

188 1972 A study of acceptance and continuation of oral contraceptives among women in a rural area. In: Sociological Evaluation of the Family Planning Programs and Research Activities in Korea. Seoul: Korean Sociological Association. Pp. 149-166.

189 LEHFELDT, H. Various

1966 ... H. GUZE: Psychological factors in contraception failure. Fertility and Sterility, 17, 110-116.

190 1967 The psychology of contraceptive failure. Medical Gynaecology and Sociology, 2, 10, 2-3.

191 LEWIT, S. Various

1973 Two years of experience with the copper-T: a research report. Studies in Family Planning, 4, 7, 171-2.

192 LIDZ, R.W. U.S.A.

1969 Emotional factors in the success of contraception. Fertility and Sterility, 20, 761-71.

193 LIPPES, J. U.S.A.
1971 ... J.G. FELDMAN: A five-year comparison of the continuation rates between women using loop D and oral contraceptives. Contraception, _3_, 5, 313-325.

194 LIU, P.T. Taiwan
1972 ... L.P. CHOW, H. ABBEY: A study of IUD retention by curve fitting. Demography, _9_, 1, 1-13.

195 1975 ... L.P. CHOW: Retention function of all segments of IUD usage: a compound distribution. Theoretical Population Biology, _8_, 1, 87-96.

196 MACCORQUODALE, D.W. Philippines
1974 Philippines physicians' influence on acceptors' selection of the IUD. Studies in Family Planning, _5_, 4, 140-143.

197 MAJUMDAR, M. India
1972 ... B.C. MULLICK, A. MOITRA, K.T. MOSLEY: Use of the oral contraceptive in urban, rural and slum areas. Studies in Family Planning, _3_, 9, 227-232.

198 MALAYSIA, FEDERATION OF FAMILY PLANNING ASSOCIATIONS Malaysia
1976 The Penang FPA: the drop-out study. FPA Newsletter, _12_,2.

199 MARKS, E.S. Various
1974 ... W. SELTZER, K.J. KROTKI: Population growth estimation: a handbook of vital statistics measurement. Population Council.

200 MARCKWARDT, A.M. Various
1974 Findings from family planning research: Latin American Supplement. Reports on Population/Family Planning, No. 12, Supplement. Pp. 8.

201 MAULDIN, W.P. Various
1967 ... D. NORTMAN, F.F. STEPHAN: Retention of IUDs: an international comparison. Studies in Family Planning, 1, 18, 1-12.

202 1975 Assessment of national family planning programs in developing countries. Studies in Family planning, 6, 2, 30-36.

203 MCALISTER, D. U.S.A.
1970 ... V. THIESSON: Prediction of the adoption and use of contraception. American Journal of Public Health, 60, 1372-1381.

204 MEASHAM, A. Colombia
1974 ... E. MARTINEZ: The role of the family in post-partum family planning acceptance. International Journal of Gynaecology and Obstetrics, 12, 2, 66-71.

205 1975 ... E. MARTINEZ: The influence of institutional and convenience factors on postpartum family planning acceptance in Medellin, Colombia. Contraception, 11, 2, 133-142.

206 1976 Self-prescription of oral contraceptives in Bogotá, Colombia. Contraception, 13, 3, 333-340.

207 MEHRA, L. India
1970 ... P.S. MOHAPATRA, B.B.L. SHARMA: A report on the oral pill pilot project clinics in India. New Delhi: Central Family Planning Institute Technical Paper No. 9. Pp. 25.

208 MICHIELUTTE, R. Costa Rica
1973 ... C.A. HANEY, C.M. COCHRANE, C.E. VINCENT: Factors associated with utilization of family planning clinics in Costa Rica. Social Biology, 20, 2, 160-172.

209 MISHELL, D.R. Various
1975 Assessing the intrauterine device. Family Planning Perspectives, 7, 3, 103-111.

210 MIYAMOTO, J. Japan
1973 Background considerations on induced abortion. International Journal of Fertility, 18, 1, 5-12.

211 MOHAPATRA, P.S. India
1971 ... et. al.: The oral pill pilot project in India. Report of the acceptor follow-up study. New Delhi: National Institute of Family Planning. Paper No. 16. Pp. 55.

212 MOON, H.S. Korea
1973 ... S.H. HAN: Use-effectiveness, extended use-effectiveness and demographic effectiveness of IUD and oral pill. Korean Institute for Family Planning. (In Korean, Tables in English). Pp. 59.

213 MOOTS, L. Taiwan
1973 ... H.C. CHEN: Preliminary report of the Taichung IUD 4 study. University of Michigan, Population Study Center; Taiwan Committee on Family Planning, Working Paper 22, Pp. 45.

214 1975 ... M.C. CHANG: Long-term use of contraceptives by IUD acceptors in Taichung, Taiwan. Studies in Family Planning, _6_, 6, 170-176.

215 MOREHEAD, J.E. U.S.A.
1975 Intrauterine device retention; a study of selected socio-psychological aspects. American Journal of Public Health, _65_, 7, 720-730.

216 MOROCCO, MINISTERE DE LA SANTE PUBLIQUE: Morocco
SERVICES CENTRAL DE LA PLANIFICATION FAMILIALE.
1972 Enquête sur la continuation des méthodes contraceptives, Vol. 3. Pp. 177.

217 1974 Enquête sur la continuation des méthodes contraceptives. Pp. 23.

218 MUNDIGO, A.I. Honduras
1970 ... J.M. STYCOS: Family planning in Honduras: A review of the national program. Ithaca: International Population Program, Cornell University.

219 1973 Honduras revisted: the clinic and its clientele. In: Clinics, Contraception and Communication, J.M. Stycos (ed.). Pp. 98-115.

220 1975 ... J.M. STYCOS: Information and evaluation in perspective: The Dominican Republic family planning program. In: The Clinic and Information Flow, J.M. Stycos (ed.). Pp. 25-58. Dominican Republic

221 MURTY, D.V.R. India
1970 ... P.S. MOHAPATRA, A.K. PRABHAKAR: An analysis of the data on IUCD cases. In: Intrauterine Contraceptive Devices, S. Roy (ed.). Proceedings of the First Seminar, Central Family Planning Institute. Pp. 281-292.

222 ONETTO, E.E. Chile
1971 ... et. al.: Clinical effectiveness of an injectable progestagen compared with IUDs evaluated by the life table method in women treated up to 33 months. In: Seventh World Congress, Fertility and Sterility, October 1971. R. Kleinmen, V.R. Pickles (eds.). Amsterdam: Excerpta Medica. Pp. 86.

223 OSTERIA, T.S. Philippines
1972 Motivational factors associated with contraceptive usage; the case of the limiters versus the spacers. Population Institute, University of the Philippines, Pp. 9.

224 PAKSHONG, D.I. Singapore
1969 ... S.M. YUNG, S.G. HU: Report of a study using a long acting injectable contraceptive, done by the family planning and population board on 750 women in Singapore. Family Planning and Population Board Paper No. 7, Pp. 8.

225 PANDIT, V.Y. India
1972 A follow-up study of the Nirodh users. Journal of Family Welfare, 18, 3, 3-11.

226 PANDOLFI, A.P. Brazil
1972 Contribuiçào ao estudio das taxas de continidade em pacientes com dispositivo intra-uterino de Lippes. Pp. 103.

227 PARDOKO, R.H. Indonesia
1972 Use effectiveness study of contraception among 1971 acceptors in East Java. National Coordinating Board for Family Planning, National Institute of Public Health, Surabaya, Pp. 38.

228 PECK, B. U.S.A.
1973 Oral contraceptive continuation/discontinuation rates. In: A Final Report on Emory University's Summer Program in Family Planning and Human Sexuality. J.D. Thompson, W.N. Long, R.A. Hatcher, J. Richardson (eds.) Pp. 20-58.

229 PEDERSEN, H.A. Various
1972 ... H.G. ELKINS, J.C. SINQUEFIELD: A simplified client record system for family planning programs. Community and Family Study Center, University of Chicago. Evaluation Manual 10. Pp. 85.

230 PENG, J.Y. Thailand
1967 ... W. ASAVESENA, S. VIMUKTANON: A pilot programme for family planning in Thailand: review of one year of operation in Potharam, 1964-5. Medical Gynecology and Sociology, 2, 7, 5-8 and 2, 8, 7-15.

231 1970 ... L.P. CHOW, L. CORSA: Medical correlates of termination of use of intrauterine contraceptive devices in Taichung. International Journal of Fertility, 15, 2, 120-6. Taiwan

232 1970 ... L.P. CHOW, L. CORSA, JR: Medical correlates of termination of use of intrauterine devices. Studies in Family Planning, 1, 60, 24-27.

233 1973 ... L.P. CHOW, S. PEDRAZA, R. AVERY: Post insertion medical symptoms and removal of the IUD in the Taiwan IUD follow-up study. Studies in Family Planning, 4, 1, 16-22.

234 1974 ... S. KEOVICHIT, R. MACINTYRE (eds.): Role of traditional birth attendants in family planning. Proceedings of a seminar held in Bangkok and Kuala Lumpur, 19-26 July, 1974. Pp. 107. Various

235 PERKIN, G.W. U.S.A.
1969 Measuring clinic performance. Family Planning Perspectives, 1, 1, 36-38.

236 PHATAK, L.V. India
1973 ... A.K. JAIN, R. CHHABRA: Post insertion contraceptive and fertility behaviour of IUCD acceptors. National Institute of Family Planning, Technical Paper No. 18. Pp. 32.

237 PHILIPPINES: U.P. POPULATION INSTITUTE. FAMILY PLANNING EVALUATION OFFICE. Philippines
1971 Preliminary continuation and pregnancy rates from follow-up surveys at three Philippine family planning clinics. Pp. 14.

238 PHILLIPS, J.F. Philippines
1974 ... Z.C. ZABLAN: Trends in first method continuation and pregnancy rates for the Philippine program over the 1970-72 period. Population Institute, University of Philippines, Research Note No. 28. Pp. 8.

239 PIERCE, A. U.S.A.
1972 ... J.M. HILLER, J. MCGUIRE: A comparison of two large scale studies on the use effectiveness of IUDs. Studies in Family Planning, 3, 9, 205-213.

240 PINCUS, G. Puerto Rico
1959 ... J. ROCK, C.R. GARCIA: Field trials with norethnynodrel as an oral contraceptive. In: Proceedings, Sixth International Conference on Planned Parenthood, New Delhi. London: IPPF. Pp. 216-230.

241 PITCHAI, S. India
1969 A follow-up of IUD cases in clinics of the Family Planning Association of India, Bombay. Publication Series No. 2. Pp. 27.

242 POPULATION INFORMATION PROGRAM, GEORGE WASHINGTON UNIVERSITY Various
1976 ... (Prepared by C.G. WUBB, R.F. BERGMAN.) Drop-outs: computer printout. Pp. 200.

243 POTTER, R.G. Jr. Various
1963 Additional measures of use-effectiveness of contraception. Milbank Memorial Fund Quarterly, 41, 400-418.

244 1966 Application of life table techniques to measurement of contraceptive effectiveness. Demography, 3, 2, 297-304.

245 1967 ... L.P. CHOW, A.K. JAIN, C.H. LEE: Expanded report on social and demographic correlates of IUCD effectiveness: The Taichung IUCD medical follow-up study. University of Michigan Population Studies Center, Pp. 69. Taiwan

246 1967 The multiple decrement life table as an approach to the measurement of use effectiveness and demographic effectiveness of contraception. In: International Union for the Scientific Study of Population, Contributed Papers, Sydney, Australia, August, 1967. Pp. 869-883. Various

247 1968 Estimating births averted in a family planning program. In: Fertility and Family Planning, S.J. Behrman, et. al. (ed.). Pp. 413-434. Taiwan

248 1968 ... R. FREEDMAN, L.P. CHOW: Taiwan's family planning program. Science, 160, 848-853. Taiwan

249 1969 Use-effectiveness of intrauterine contraception as a problem in competing risks. In: Family Planning in Taiwan: An Experiment in Social Change. R. Freedman, J.Y. Takeshita (eds.) Pp. 458-484.

250 1969 ... L.P. CHOW, A.K. JAIN, C.H. LEE: Effectiveness of intrauterine contraception: termination levels and correlates. In: Family Planning in Taiwan: An Experiment in Social Change. R. Freedman et. al. (eds.) Pp. 241-279.

251 1970 ... A.K. JAIN, B. MCCANN: Net delay of next conception by contraception: a highly simplified case. Population Studies, 24, 2, 173-191.

252 1970 ... B. MCCANN, J.M. SAKODA: Selective fecundability and contraceptive effectiveness. Milbank Memorial Fund Quarterly, 48, 91-102. Various

253 1971 Inadequacy of a one method family planning program. Studies in Family Planning, 2, 1, 1-6. (Also in Social Biology, 18, 1, 1-9). Various

254 1972 ... P.S.K. CHI, J.M. SAKODA: Number and mean age of acceptors and users as related to programme duration. Population Studies, 26, 2, 307-316.

255 1975 ... R.C. AVERY: Use-effectiveness of contraception. In: Measuring the effect of family planning programs on fertility. C. Chandrasekaran, A.I. Hermalin (eds.) Pp. 133-208. Various

256 POTTS, M. Colombia, Antigua
1973 Contraceptive distribution in Colombia and Antigua. IPPF, London Pp. 26.

257 PURI, A.P. India
1970 ... B. MISHRA: Longitudinal study of oral contraceptive acceptors. Family Planning News, 11, 1, 2-5.

258 RAMAKRISHNAN, S.A. India
1971 ... N. SAMPOORNAM: A case study of the drop-outs in the oral contraceptive pilot project, Madras. The Journal of Family Welfare, 17 4, 44-56.

259 RAO, A.P. — India
1972 Five year follow-up study of Lippes loop. Antiseptic, 69, 2, 109.

260 RAO, H. — India
1971 ... R. VASANTHINI, B.A. SATYANARAYANA CHAR.: A study of abortion cases in Bangalore City Hospitals. Journal of Family Welfare, 18, 2, 81-87.

261 REYNOLDS, J. — Various
1970 ... R. RAMAPRASAD: A method for estimating future caseloads. Manuals for Evaluation of Family Planning and Population Programs. Number 3. International Institute for the Study of Human Reproduction. Pp. 35.

262 1971 Family Planning drop-outs in Trinidad and Tobago. Social and Economic Studies, 20, 2, 176-187. — Trinidad and Tobago

263 1972 Evaluation of family planning program performance: A critical review. Demography, 9, 1, 69-85. — Various

264 1972 ... M.E. ROVIRA: Estimación de casos activos y cobertura del programa nacional de planificación familiar en Costa Rica en 1971. San José: Universidad de Costa Rica. Centro de Estudios Sociales y de Población. Pp. 21. — Costa Rica

265 RIDER, R.V. — Pakistan
1966 ... et. al.: Use of the intra-uterine device in rural West Pakistan. Demography, 3, 2, 332-42.

266 ROGERS, E.M. Various
1975 ... D.S. SOLOMON: Traditional midwives for family planning communication in Asia. Honolulu: East-West Communications Institute.

267 1975 ... D.S. SOLOMON: Traditional midwives and family planning in Asia. Studies in Family Planning, 6, 5, 126-133.

268 ROMM, F.J. U.S.A.
1975 ... P.S. ARMSTRONG, A.P. PRIOR: A comparison of program and contraceptive use continuation rates in a family planning clinic. American Journal of Public Health, 65, 7, 695-99.

269 ROSENFIELD, A.G. Thailand
1971 Family Planning: an expanded role for paramedical personnel. American Journal of Obstetrics and Gynecology, 110, 7, 1030-1039.

270 ROSENFIELD, A.G. Thailand
1972 ... C. LIMCHAROEN: Auxiliary midwife prescription of oral contraceptives: An experimental project in Thailand. American Journal of Obstetrics and Gynecology, 114, 7, 942-949.

271 1972 ... S. VARAKAMIN: The postpartum approach to family planning experience: in Thailand. American Journal of Obstetrics and Gynecology, 113, 1, 1-13.

No.	Author / Year	Reference	Country
272	ROSS, J.A. 1968	... F.F. STEPHAN, W.B. WATSON: A handbook for service statistics in family planning programs. The Population Council. Pp. 147.	Various
273	1970	... et. al.: Korea/Taiwan 1969: report on the national family planning program. Studies in Family Planning, 1, 54, 1-16.	Korea Taiwan
274	1972	... J.E. FORREST: Program effects upon fertility. In: Statistical Problems in Population Research, N. Keyfitz (ed.).	Various
275	1972	... A. GERMAIN, J.E. FORREST, J. VAN GINNEKEN: Findings from family planning research. Reports on Population/Family Planning, No. 12. Pp. 47.	
276	RYDER, N.B. 1972	Time series of Pill and IUD use: United States, 1961-1970. Studies in Family Planning, 3, 10, 233-240	U.S.A.
277	1972	... C.F. WESTOFF: Wanted and unwanted fertility in the United States: 1965 and 1970. In: Demographic and Social Aspects of Population Growth, C.F. Westoff, R. Parks, Jr., (eds.). Research Reports of the U.S. Commission on Population Growth and the American Future, Vol. I. Pp. 467-488.	
278	1973	Contraceptive failure in the United States. Family Planning Perspectives, 5, 3, 133-142.	

279 SADASHIVAIAH, K. India
1971 ... R. CHRISTOPHER, S.G. SAMPATH IYANGAR, A.S. RAMESH: A report on the oral pill project of Mission Hospitals in India. Family Planning Project of the Christian Medical Association of India. Technical Paper 10, Pp. 24.

280 1971 ... M.S. SUBBA RAO, J.S. SIMHA: The oral pill program: a summary of preliminary findings. Journal of the Christian Medical Association of India, 46, 4, 208-13.

281 1973 ... M.S. SUBBHA RAO: Evaluation of intrauterine contraception in selected mission hospitals in India. Journal of Biosocial Science, 5, 3, 377-391.

282 1974 ... A.S. RAMESH, J.S. SIMHA: A retrospective study of the oral pill acceptors in the member mission hospitals of the southern region. Paper prepared for a seminar on family planning research studies held at the Institute for Rural Health and Family Planning Gandhigram, Madurai District, Tamilnadu, India. January 3-5, 1974. Pp. 23.

283 SADIK, N. Various
1968 Assessment of acceptance, use and use-effectiveness of contraceptive methods. In: U.N. Economic Commission for Asia and the Far East. Expert Group on Assessment of Acceptance and Use-effectiveness of Family Planning Methods. Bangkok, Thailand, June 11-21. New York: U.N. Economic and Social Council. Pp. 15.

284 SAKSENA, D.N. India
1973 ... H. BHENDE: Continuation rates, complaints and reasons for discontinuance relating to contraceptive pills: an Indian experience. Indian Journal of Public Health, 17, 1, 3.

285 SANDBERG, E.D. Various
1971 ... R.I. JACOBS: Psychology of the misuse and rejection of contraception. American Journal of Obstetrics and Gynecology, 110, 2, 227-239.

286 SANDHU, S.K. India
1970 ... K.S. BHARDWAJ: Follow-up study of dropped cases in Paharganj area. New Delhi: Central Family Planning Institute, Monograph Series 15. Pp. 78.

287 SARRAM, M. Iran
1975 ... A.A. PAYDARFAR, L.P. COLE: Acceptance, continuation and termination of IUD users: a pilot study among Shirazi women. Iran Population Studies Program, Carolina Population Center. Pp. 20.

288 SATTERTHWAITE, A.P. Puerto Rico
1966 Oral contraceptives. In: Family Planning and Population Programs. B. Berelson, et. al. (eds.). Pp. 411-424.

289 SAXTON, G.A. Uganda
1969 ... M.C. PIKE: Long term effectiveness and acceptability of IUCDs in Uganda. East African Medical Journal, 46, 2, 107-120.

290 SCRIMSHAW, S.C.M. Ecuador
1976 Women's modesty: one barrier to the use of family planning clinics in Ecuador. In: J.F. Marshall, S. Polgar (eds.). Culture, Natality and Family Planning. Pp. 167-183.

291 SEAL, K.C. India
1974 ... P.P. TALWAR: Impact of some patterns of spacing on fertility: a case study of India. Journal of Family Welfare, _21_, 2, 13.

292 SEAR, A.M. U.S.A.
1973 Clinic discontinuation and contraceptive need. Family Planning Perspectives, _5_, 2, 80-88.

293 1974 ... M.N. TURNER: Factors associated with short-term oral contraceptive discontinuation. Family Planning Perspectives, _6_, 4, 230-33.

294 SELMAN, P. U.K.
1973 ... C. STEPHENS: Missed appointments at a family clinic. Journal of Biosocial Science, _5_, 4, 421-442.

295 SHAPIRO, P. U.K.
1962 The unplanned children. New Society, _5_, 19-23.

296 SHIN, H.S. Korea
1967 Extended clinical trial with IUD in Korea: fourth progress report. Department of Obstetrics and Gynecology. Seoul National University. Pp. 18.

297 1970 ... S.W. KIM: Use-effectiveness of the IUD in Korea. In: Population and Family Planning in the Republic of Korea, Vol. 1. Seoul Ministry of Health and Social Affairs. Pp. 91-107.

298 SIASSI, I. Iran
1972 The psychiatrist's role in family planning. American Journal of Psychiatry, 129, 1, 80-85.

299 SIEGEL, E. U.S.A.
1971 ... et. al.: Continuation of contraception by low income women: a one year follow-up. American Journal of Public Health, 61, 9, 1886-1898.

300 SIMHA, J.S. India
1972 ... A.S. RAMESH: Comparative study of oral acceptors in the three member missions of Mysore State. Journal of the Christian Medical Association of India, 47, 10, 513-518.

301 SIMMONS, A.B. Colombia
1973 Information campaigns and the growth of family planning in Colombia. In: Clinics, Contraception and Communication, J.M. Stycos (ed.) Pp. 116-171.

302 SINGH, B.R. India
1972 ... S.C. BAGCHI: A study of the effectiveness of intrauterine devices in Allahabad. Indian Journal of Public Health, 16, 2, 47.

303 SINQUEFIELD, J.C. Various
1973 Single and multiple decrement life table procedures for the analysis of the use-effectiveness of contraception. Family Planning Research and Evaluation Manual, No. 8. Community and Family Study Center, University of Chicago. Pp. 131.

304 1974 A social-psychological study of resistance to family planning in rural Alabama. Chicago: University of Chicago: Community and Family Study Center. Pp. 136. U.S.A.

305 SIVIN, I Various
1971 Fertility decline and contraceptive use in the international postpartum and family planning program. Studies in Family Planning, 2, 12, 248-256.

306 1974 Contraception and fertility change in the International Postpartum Program. Technical Assistance Division. The Population Council. Pp. 98.

307 1976 A comparison of the Copper T-200 and the Lippes loop in four countries. Studies in Family Planning, 7, 4, 115-122.

308 SLAVIN, S.L. Barbados
1974 ... R.E. BILSBORROW: The Barbados family planning association and fertility decline in Barbados. Studies in Family Planning, 5, 10, 325-332.

309 SLOCUMB, J.C. U.S.A.
1975 ... C.L. ODOROFF, S.J. KUNITZ: The use-effectiveness of two contraceptive methods in a Navajo population: the problem of program drop-outs. American Journal of Obstetrics and Gynecology, 122, 6, 717-726.

310 SNOWDEN, R. U.K.
1971 Social factors in use and effectiveness of the IUD. Ph. D. Thesis, University of Exeter.

311 1975 ... P. ECKSTEIN, D. HAWKINS: Social and medical factors in the use and effectiveness of IUDs. Journal of Biosocial Science, 5, 2, 31-50.

312 SOEGENG, W. Indonesia
1973 Results of a study of use-effectiveness of contraceptive methods: Bali, 1971-2. Denpasar: National Family Planning Coordinating Board.

313 SOETEDJO, M. Indonesia
1972 ... J. CLINTON: Trends in contraceptive use: the Indonesian experience. Technical Report Series. Monograph Number 4, Pp. 19.

314 1973 Contraceptive trends in Indonesia's developing family planning program. Technical Report Series. Monograph Number 5, Pp. 25.

315 SOMBOONSUK, A. Thailand
1973 ... A.G. ROSENFIELD: Experiences with the Lippes loop, 1965-71. International Journal of Gynaecology and Obstetrics, 11, 1, 16-24.

316 SONI, K. India
1976 ... et. al.: Characteristics of women seeking medical termination of pregnancy. Journal of Family Welfare. <u>22</u>, 3, 51-61.

317 SPEIDEL, J.J. U.S.A.
1970 ... L. WEINER: Continuance of family planning in a Health Department Clinic. American Journal of Obstetrics and Gynecology, <u>108</u>, 7, 1134-1140.

318 SRI LANKA: FAMILY PLANNING EVALUATION UNIT Sri Lanka
1969 Oral contraceptive follow-up survey: selected MOH areas, Kurunegala. Evaluation Report 5. Pp. 5.

319 STYCOS, J.M. (ed.) Various
1973 Clinics, contraception and communication: evaluation studies of family planning programs in four Latin American countries. Pp. 207.

320 1975 (ed). The clinic and information flow. Pp. 174.

321 SUGATHAN, T.N. India
1974 ... B.B.L. SHARMA: Clinical services and follow-up of oral pill acceptance. Journal of Population Research. <u>1</u>, 1, 59-69.

322 SULLIVAN, J. Indonesia
1976 ... H. SUYONO, W. BAHRAWI, A. HARTOADI: Contraceptive use-effectiveness in Mojokerto Regency, Indonesia: A comparison of regular program and special drive acceptors. Studies in Family Planning, <u>7</u>, 7, 188-196.

323 SUVANAVEJH, C. Thailand
1970 Factors affecting the continuation of contraceptive use. Student Paper: School of Public Health, University of North Carolina. Pp. 14.

324 SWARAJYALAKSHMI, B. India
1970 ... K.R. ANAYSUA: A follow-up study of IUD cases in Visakhapatnam District. Journal of Family Welfare, 17, 2, 9-19.

325 SWEENY, H.C. India
1970 Topical investigation and analysis of rehabilitating the IUD in South Asia. Research Triangle Institute, Research Triangle Park, North Carolina. Pp. 40.

326 TAIWAN: INSTITUTE OF FAMILY PLANNING Taiwan
1970 A selective bibliography of published studies about population in Taiwan. Taiwan Population Studies, Working Paper Number 8, Pp. 8.

327 TAIWAN: PROVINCIAL DEPARTMENT OF HEALTH, COMMITTEE ON FAMILY PLANNING, TAIPEI. Taiwan
1970 Family planning reference book, V.3. loop acceptance, 1969. Pp. 205.

328 1970 Family planning reference book, V.4. pill acceptance, 1969, Pp. 78.

329 TAIWAN: THE CHINESE CENTRE FOR INTERNATIONAL TRAINING IN FAMILY PLANNING. Taiwan
1972 Taiwan's family planning in charts. 5th ed. Taichung, Pp. 61.

330 TAKESHITA, J.Y. Malaysia
1970 ... T.B. ANN, L.M. VERBRUGGE: West Malaysia: 1969 family planning acceptor follow-up survey. Studies in Family Planning, 1, 51, 18-23.

331 THAILAND: NATIONAL FAMILY PLANNING PROJECT MINISTRY OF PUBLIC HEALTH. Thailand

1971 Family planning in Thailand, 1965-70, Pp. 28; 1965-71, Pp. 35.

332 TIETZE, C. Various

1951 ... S.R. POLIAKOFF, J. ROCK: The clinical effectiveness of the rhythm method of contraception. Fertility and Sterility, 2, 444-50.

333 1960 The condom as a contraceptive. The National Committee on Maternal Health. Washington D.C. Pp. 39.

334 1960 Probability of pregnancy resulting from a single unprotected coitus. Fertility and Sterility, 11, 5, 485-488.

335 1962 ... R.G. POTTER, JR.: Current opinion, re-evaluation, statistical evaluation of the rhythm method. American Journal of Obstetrics and Gynecology, 84, 692-8.

336 1965 Effectiveness and acceptability of IUD devices. American Journal of Public Health, 55, 1874-9.

337 1966 Intrauterine contraception: research report. Studies in Family Planning, 1, 12, 10-13.

338 1967 Intrauterine contraception: recommended procedures for data analysis. Studies in Family Planning, 1, 18, (supplement), 1-16.

339 1967 ... S. LEWIT: Comparison of three contraceptive methods: diaphragm with jelly or cream, vaginal foam, and jelly/cream alone. Journal of Sex Research, 3, 4, 295-311. U.S.A.

340 1968 ... S. LEWIT: Effectiveness and continuation of contraception: problems of evaluation. In: U.N. Economic Commission for Asia and the Far East. Expert Group on Assessment of Acceptance and Use-Effectiveness of Family Planning Methods, Bangkok, Thailand, June 11-21. Vol. 1. New York, U.N.E.S.C.O. Pp. 19. Various

341 1968 ... S. LEWIT: Statistical evaluation of contraceptive methods: use-effectiveness and extended use-effectiveness. Demography, 5, 2, 931-940.

342 1970 Fertility after discontinuation of intrauterine and oral contraception. In: World Congress on Fertility and Sterility. Tel Aviv, May 20-27, 1968. Pp. 237-241. Jerusalem, Israel. Israel Academy of Sciences and Humanities.

343 1970 ... S. LEWIT: Evaluation of intra-uterine devices: ninth progress report of the Co-operative Statistical Program. Studies in Family Planning, 1, 55, 1-40.

344 1970 ... S. LEWIT: Statistical evaluation of contraceptive methods: use-effectiveness and extended use-effectiveness. Follow-up and appendix to article by same title appearing in Demography 1968. Paper presented at Workshop on Evaluation of Family Planning Programmes, Santiago, January 1970. CELADE, Series D, No. 55. Pp. 27.

345 TIETZE, C. Various
1971 ... S. LEWIT: Use-effectiveness of oral and intrauterine contraception. Fertility and Sterility, 22, 8, 508-13.

346 1972 ... S. LEWIT: Comparison of the Copper T and loop D: a research report. Studies in Family Planning, 3, 11, 277-8.

347 1973 ... S. LEWIT: Recommended procedures for the statistical evaluation of intra-uterine contraception. Studies in Family Planning, 4, 2, 35-41.

348 1975 ... M.C. MURSTEIN: Induced abortion: 1975 handbook. Reports on Population/Family Planning No. 14 (Second Edition). Pp. 75.

349 TISSAINAYAGAM, M.B.J. Barbados
1973 Follow-up survey of pill acceptors (1970-1) with special emphasis on 'discontinuing users'. Barbados Family Planning Association. Pp.18.

350 TUNISIA: OFFICE NATIONAL DU PLANNING FAMILIAL ET DE LA POPULATION Tunisia
1973 Enquête nationale sur la continuation des méthodes contraceptives, 2 vols. Pp. 138, 119.

351 TUNISIA: SERVICES DES STATISTIQUES, RECHERCHE ET EVALUATION
1971 Statistiques de Programme national: post-partum et post-abortion pour l'anee 1970. Tunis: Ministere De La Santé Publique.

352 TURKEY: MINISTRY OF HEALTH Turkey
1971 Turkish IUD retention survey, 1969. Ministry of Health, Population Planning Publication, No. 408. Pp. 65.

353 UNITED NATIONS: ECONOMIC COMMISSION FOR ASIA AND THE FAR EAST Various
1968 Assessment of acceptance and effectiveness of family planning methods: report of an expert group. Bangkok, Thailand, June 11-21. Series No. 4. Pp. 68.

354 1968 Problems arising in defining acceptance, use and effectiveness in the evaluation of family planning programmes. In: U.N. Economic Commission for Asia and the Far East. Expert Group on Assessment of Acceptance and Use-effectiveness of Family Planning Methods, Bangkok, Thailand, June 11-21, 1968. Vol. 1. Pp.19.

355 1969 Evaluation of Family Planning Programmes. Asian Population Studies No. 5.

356 VARAKAMIN, S. Thailand
1971 Preliminary report on the follow-up surveys of acceptors of family planning services, March-April 1970. Bangkok: Ministry of Public Health.

357 VERMA, V. India
1972 ... S.C. BAGCHI: Acceptability and use-effectiveness of an oral contraceptive in a rural area. Indian Journal of Medical Research, 60, 8, 1242-1250.

358 VIEL, B. India

1970 The effect of a contraceptive program on induced abortion. International Journal of Gynaecology and Obstetrics. 8, 2 pt., 714-717.

359 VIMUKTANON, S. Thailand
1971 ... A.G. ROSENFIELD: An IUD follow-up study in Potharam, Thailand. Studies in Family Planning, 2, 8, 166-170.

360 WAN, F.K. Singapore
1971 ... S.T. QUAH: Singapore: a study of clinic continuation rates. Studies in Family Planning, 2, 12, 257-258.

361 1975 ... A.J. CHEN, J. TAN: Oral contraceptive continuation rates in the Singapore national program, 1962-1972. Studies in Family Planning, 6, 1, 17-21.

362 WARD, A. U.K.
1971 Why do family planning patients drop out? Journal of Biosocial Science 3, 3, 301-308.

363 WELLER, R.H. U.S.A.
1976 Number and timing failures among legitimate births in the United States: 1968, 1969, 1972. Family Planning Perspectives, 8, 3, 111-116.

364 WELLS, H.B. Various
1969 Design of follow-up surveys for assessing continuation of use of contraceptive methods. Chapel Hill, N.C.: Carolina Population Center. Paper prepared for the Seminar on Evaluation of Family Planning Programs, U.N. ECAFE, 24 Nov. - 12 Dec. 1969. Pp. 44.

365 WESTOFF, C.F. U.S.A.
1968 ... N.B. RYDER: Duration of use of oral contraception in the United States, 1960-65. Public Health Reports, 83, 277-287.

366 1975 ... E.F. JONES: Discontinuation of the pill and the IUD in the United States: 1960-1970. Journal of Neuropathology and Experimental Neurology. 42, 4, 384-390.

367 WEST PAKISTAN RESEARCH AND EVALUATION CENTER Pakistan
1968 IUD retention in West Pakistan: a report of experience in the first eighteen months of the National Family Planning Program. July 1965 - December 1966.

368 WISHIK, S.M. Various
1968 Indexes for measurement of amount of contraception practice. Paper presented at a meeting of Expert Group on Assessment of Acceptance and Use-Effectiveness of Family Planning Methods, United Nations Economic Commission for Asia and the Far East, Bangkok, Thailand, June 11-21. Pp. 15.

369 1974 ... N. SADIK: Approaches to measurement of the impact of family planning programs on the prevalence of contraceptive practice. In: International Population Conference, Liege, 1973. Vol. 2. International Union for the Scientific Study of Population. Pp. 225-231.

370 WOLFERS, D. Singapore
1969 The demographic effects of a contraceptive programme. Population Studies, 23, 111-141.

371 1970 ... (ed.): Postpartum intrauterine contraception in Singapore. Amsterdam: Excerpta Medica Foundation. Pp. 193.

372 1970 ... S.S. RATNAM: Follow-up study of inserted women. In: Postpartum Intrauterine Contraception in Singapore. D. Wolfers, (ed.) Pp. 105-119.

373 WORTH, G. Korea
1971 ... et. al.: Korea/Taiwan 1970: Report on the national family planning programs. Studies in Family Planning, 2, 3, 57-69.

374 WORTMAN, J. Various
1976 Barrier methods: the diaphragm and other intravaginal barriers; a review. Population Reports, 4, 57-76.

375 WRIGHT, N.H. Various
1969 Natural history of contraceptive practice among post-partum loop acceptors. Obstetrics and Gynaecology, 33, 3, 361-369.

376 1972 International postpartum program: analysis of performance 1970-1971. Studies in Family Planning, 3, 12, 305-308.

377 1973 ... T. PERERA. Ceylon: Continuing practice of contraception by acceptors of oral contraceptives and intrauterine devices in a field program. Bulletin of the World Health Organization, 48, 639-47. Sri Lanka

378 1975 Sri Lanka: the impact of allowing paramedical prescription and resupply of oral contraceptives. Studies in Family Planning, 6, 4, 102-5.

379 XENOS, C. Mauritius
1970 Mauritius. Country Profiles. New York: Population Council: Inter-National Institute for the Study of Human Reproduction. Columbia University.

380 YANG, J.M. Korea
1968 ... et. al.: Study on the acceptability and effectiveness of an oral contraceptive among IUD drop-outs in rural Korea. Seoul: Department of Preventive Medicine and Public Health, Yonsei University.

381 1968 ... et. al.: Improving access to the IUD: experiments in Koyang, Korea. Studies in Family Planning, _1_, 27, 4-11.

382 1972 Studies in family planning and related programs in rural Korea. In: Sociological Evaluation of the Family Planning Programs and Research Activities in Korea. Seoul: Korean Sociological Association, Pp. 111-35.

383 ZABLAN, Z.C. Philippines
n.d. IUCD Retention rates among family planning patients at the Philippines General Hospital. Population Institute, University of the Philippines, Pp. 21.

384 ZABLAN, Z.C. Philippines
1974 The relative importance of accessibility factors in family planning clinic utilization: national acceptor survey, Philippines, 1972. Manila: Population Institute, University of the Philippines, Research Note No. 21. Pp. 12.

385 ZATUCHNI, G.I. Various
1970 Postpartum family planning: a report on the international program. Population Council, Pp. 508.

386 ZEIGHAMI, E. Iran
1976 ... et. al.: Effectiveness of the Iranian auxiliary midwife in IUD insertion. Studies in Family Planning, 7, 9, 261-263.

ADDENDUM

387 BAILEY, J. Colombia
1976 ... C. MEASHAM, M. UMANA: Fertility and contraceptive practice: Bogotá 1964-1974. Studies in Family Planning 7, 9, 249-260.

388 JAIN, A.K. Taiwan
1977 ... B. MOOTS: Fecundability following the discontinuation of IUD use among Taiwanese women. Journal of Biosocial Science 9, 2, 137-151.

389 1977 ... I. SIVIN: Life table analysis of IUD's: Problems and recommendations. Studies in Family Planning 8, 2, 26-47.

390 LARSEN, T.B. General
1977 Record-keeping for contraceptive delivery systems. Evaluation Guide No. 3., International Planned Parenthood Federation. Pp.35.

391 MODE, C.J. General
1977 ... et. al.: Methodological issues underlying multiple decrement life table analysis. Demography 14, 1, 87-96.

392 RYDER, N.B. General
1976 The predictability of fertility planning status. Studies in Family Planning 7, 11, 294-307.

393 SU, I.H. Taiwan
1976 ... L.P. CHOW: Induced abortion and contraceptive practice: the experience in Taiwan. Studies in Family Planning 7, 8, 224-230.

394 TREADWAY, R.C. Iran
1976 ... R.W. GILLESPIE, M. LOGHMANI: The model family planning project in Isfahan, Iran. Studies in Family Planning 7, 11, 308-321.

395 VESSEY, M. United Kingdom
1976 ... et. al.: A long term follow-up study of women using different methods of contraception - an interim report. Journal of Biosocial Science, 8, 4, 373-427.

396 YEN, C.H. Taiwan
1976 Village and household availability of contraception: the Taiwan experience. In: J. Gardner, R.J. Wolff (eds.) Village and Household Availability of Contraceptives: South East Asia. Battelle Population Study Center, Pp. 67-76.